Computers and Medicine

Helmuth F. Orthner, *Series Editor*

Springer

New York
Berlin
Heidelberg
Barcelona
Budapest
Hong Kong
London
Milan
Paris
Santa Clara
Singapore
Tokyo

Computers and Medicine

Homer R. Warner
Dean K. Sorenson
Omar Bouhaddou

Knowledge Engineering
in Health Informatics

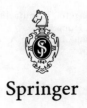

Springer

Homer R. Warner, M.D., Ph.D.
Former Chairman and Professor
  Emeritus
Department of Medical Informatics
University of Utah School of
  Medicine
Salt Lake City, UT 84132, USA

Dean K. Sorenson, Ph.D.
Assistant Research Professor
Department of Medical Informatics
University of Utah School of Medicine
Salt Lake City, UT 84132, USA

Omar Bouhaddou, Ph.D.
Chief Knowledge Engineer
Mosby Consumer Health
Salt Lake City, UT 84109, USA

Series Editor
Helmuth F. Orthner, Ph.D.
Professor of Medical Informatics
University of Utah Health Sciences
  Center
Salt Lake City, UT 84132, USA

Library of Congress Cataloging-in-Publication Data
Warner, Homer R., 1922–
    Knowledge engineering in health informatics / by Homer R. Warner,
Dean K. Sorenson, Omar Bouhaddou.
        p.   cm.—(Computers and medicine)
    Includes bibliographical references and index.
    ISBN 0-387-94901-1 (hardcover: alk. paper)
    1. Medicine–Decision making—Data processing.   2. Expert systems (Computer
science)   3. Knowledge acquisition (Expert systems)   4. Medical informatics.
    5. Diagnosis–Data processing.   I. Sorenson, Dean K., 1947–   .   II. Bouhaddou,
Omar.   III. Title.   IV. Series: Computers and medicine (New York, N.Y.)
    R859.7.D52W37   1997
    610′.285′633—dc20   96-44233

Printed on acid-free paper.

Production managed by Victoria Evarretta; manufacturing supervised by Jeffrey Taub.
Typeset by Best-set Typesetter Ltd., Hong Kong.
Printed and bound by Braun-Brumfield, Inc., Ann Arbor, MI.
Printed in the United States of America.

9 8 7 6 5 4 3 2 1

ISBN 0-387-94901-1 Springer-Verlag New York Berlin Heidelberg   SPIN 10552855

Series Preface

This monograph series is intended to provide medical information scientists, health care administrators, physicians, nurses, other health care providers, and computer science professionals with successful examples and experiences of computer applications in health care settings. Through these computer applications, we attempt to show what is effective and efficient, and hope to provide guidance on the acquisition or design of medical information systems so that costly mistakes can be avoided.

Health care provider organizations such as hospitals and clinics are experiencing large demands for clinical information because of a transition from a "fee-for-service" to a "capitation-based" health care economy. This transition changes the way health care services are being paid for. Previously, nearly all health care services were paid for by insurance companies after the services were performed. Today, many procedures need to be preapproved and many charges for clinical services must be justified to the insurance plans. Ultimately, in a totally capitated system, the more patient care services are provided per patient, the less profitable the health care provider organization will be. Clearly, the financial risks have shifted from the insurance carriers to the health care provider organizations. For hospitals and clinics to assess these financial risks, management needs to know what services are to be provided and how to reduce them without impacting the quality of care. The balancing act of reducing costs but maintaining health care quality and patient satisfaction requires accurate information about the clinical services. The only way this information can be collected cost effectively is through the automation of the health care process itself. Unfortunately, current health information systems are not comprehensive enough and their level of integration is low and primitive at best. There are too many "islands" even within single health care provider organizations.

With the rapid advance of digital communications technologies and the acceptance of standard interfaces, these "islands" can be bridged to satisfy most information needs of health care professionals and management. In addition, the migration of health information systems to client/server computer architectures allows us to reengineer the user interface to become more functional, pleasant, and also responsive. Eventually, we hope, the clinical workstation will become the tool that health care providers use interactively without intermediary data entry support.

Computer-based information systems provide more timely and legible information than traditional paper-based systems. In addition, medical information systems can monitor the process of health care and improve quality of patient care by providing decision support for diagnosis or therapy, clinical reminders for follow-up care, warnings about adverse drug interactions, alerts to questionable treatment or deviations from clinical protocols, and more. The complexity of the health care workplace requires a rich set of requirements for health information systems. Further, the systems must respond quickly to user interactions and queries to facilitate and not impede the work of health care professionals. Because of this and the requirement for a high level of security, these systems can be classified as very complex and, from a developer's perspective, also as "risky" systems.

Information technology is advancing at an accelerated pace. Instead of waiting for 3 years for a new generation of computer hardware, we are now confronted with new computing hardware every 18 months. The forthcoming changes in the telecommunications industry will be revolutionary. Within the next 5 years, or so, new digital communications technologies, such as the Integrated Services Digital Network (ISDN), Asynchronous Data Subscriber Loop (ADSL) technologies, and very high speed local area networks using efficient cell switching protocols (e.g., ATM), will change not only the architecture of our information systems but also the way we work and manage health care institutions.

The software industry constantly tries to provide tools and productive development environments for the design, implementation, and maintenance of information systems. Still, the development of information systems in medicine is an art, and the tools we use are often self-made and crude. One area that needs desperate attention is the interaction of health care providers with the computer. While the user interface needs improvement and the emerging graphical user interfaces form the basis for such improvements, the most important criterion is to provide relevant and accurate information without drowning the physician in too much (irrelevant) data.

To develop an effective clinical system requires an understanding of what is to be done and how to do it, and an understanding of how to integrate information systems into an operational health care environment. Such knowledge is rarely found in any one individual; all systems described in this monograph series are the work of teams. The size of these teams is usually small, and the composition is heterogeneous, i.e., health professionals, computer and communications scientists and engineers, statisticians, epidemiologists, etc. The team members are usually dedicated to working together over long periods of time, sometimes spanning decades.

Clinical information systems are dynamic systems, their functionality constantly changing because of external pressures and administrative changes in health care institutions. Good clinical information systems will and should change the operational mode of patient care, which, in turn, should affect the functional requirements of the information systems. This interplay requires that medical information systems be based on architectures that allow them to be adapted rapidly and with minimal expense. It also requires a willingness by management of the health care institution to adjust its operational procedures, and, most of all, to provide end-user education in the use of information technology. While medical information systems should be functionally integrated, these systems should also be modular so that incremental upgrades, additions, and deletions of modules can be done to match the pattern of capital resources and investments available to an institution.

We are building medical information systems just as automobiles were built early in this century, i.e., in an ad hoc manner that disregards even existent standards. Although technical standards addressing computer and communications technologies are necessary, they are insufficient. We still need to develop conventions and agreements, and perhaps a few regulations that address the principal use of medical information in computer and communication systems. Standardization allows the mass production of low-cost parts that can be used to build more complex structures. What exactly are these parts in medical information systems? We need to identify them, classify them, describe them, publish their specifications, and, most importantly, use them in real health care settings. We must be sure that these parts are useful and cost effective even before we standardize them.

Clinical research, health services research, and medical education will benefit greatly when controlled vocabularies are used more widely in the practice of medicine. For practical reasons, the medical profession has developed numerous classifications, nomenclatures, dictionary codes, and thesauri (e.g., ICD, CPT, DSM-III, SNOMED, COSTAR dictionary codes, BAIK thesaurus terms, and MESH terms). The collection of these terms represents a considerable amount of clinical activities, a large portion of the health care business, and access to our recorded knowledge. These terms and codes form the glue that links the practice of medicine with the business of medicine. They also link the practice of medicine with the literature of medicine, with further links to medical research and education. Because information systems are more efficient in retrieving information when controlled vocabularies are used in large databases, the attempt to unify and build bridges between these coding systems is a great example of unifying the field of medicine and health care by providing and using medical informatics tools. The Unified Medical Language System (UMLS) project of the National Library of Medicine, NIH, in Bethesda, Maryland, is an example of such an effort.

The purpose of this series is to capture the experience of medical informatics teams that have successfully implemented and operated medical information systems. We hope the individual books in this series will contribute to the evolution of medical informatics as a recognized professional discipline. We are at the threshold where there is not just the need but already the momentum and interest in the health care and computer science communities to identify and recognize the new discipline called Medical Informatics.

I would like to thank the editors of Springer-Verlag New York for the opportunity to edit this series. Also, many thanks to the present and past departmental chairmen who allowed me to spend time on this activity: William S. Yamamoto, M.D., and Thomas E. Piemme, M.D., of the Department of Computer Medicine at George Washington University Medical Center in Washington, D.C., and Homer R. Warner, M.D., Ph.D., and Reed M. Gardner, Ph.D., of the Department of Medical Informatics at the University of Utah Health Sciences Center in Salt Lake City, Utah. Last, but not least, I thank all authors and editors of this monograph series for contributing to the practice and theory of Medical Informatics.

HELMUTH F. ORTHNER

Preface

This book was conceived to meet three primary objectives. First, to make known the principles and methods of knowledge engineering developed over nine years of experience with the Iliad diagnostic medical expert system. Second, to provide a textbook to be used for a course in knowledge engineering in a medical informatics curriculum. Third, to provide "physician hackers" and other neophytes with the necessary information and software tools to develop their own expert systems.

We have attempted to keep the presentation generic, but have also tried to use many examples. We have used examples from the Iliad medical expert system throughout the book because that is the system we are most familiar with. Other well-known comprehensive medical expert systems include QMR and DXplain. And, there are many other more specialized systems that have been reported, both in the U.S. and elsewhere. Many systems attest to the need that has been recognized and to the potential usefulness that many have tried to fill. The field is rapidly changing for a number of reasons, e.g., many disciplines are involved, funding and management of healthcare in general is in a rapid state of flux, and the underlying basic science that explains disease etiology and drives the development of new therapies is rapidly changing. There is no perfect medical expert system; each has strengths and weaknesses. Likewise, there is no knowledge engineering method that has been proved to be superior to all others.

It is our hope that readers of this book will come to appreciate the power and sophistication of the Iliad expert system. It is also our hope that many of the principles described here will be applicable to other medical expert systems and to other knowledge engineering environments. We have attempted here to formulate general concepts and principles where possible and to point up potential problems in the knowledge engineering process necessary to build medical expert systems. The methods proposed here are not necessarily the only methods or the best methods for any given situation.

HOMER R. WARNER
DEAN K. SORENSON
OMAR BOUHADDOU

Acknowledgments

We would like to acknowledge the contributions of others to this work.

Hong Yu, M.S., has managed the Iliad dictionary and the knowledge authoring process, and authored Appendix 3 ("Using the Iliad knowledge engineering tools").

Homer Warner, Jr., M.S., had a leadership role in managing the development of the Iliad software and contributing to the commercial development of the program.

Peter Haug, M.D., has been involved in Iliad development since its inception and has taken a leading role in teaching medical informatics students how to do knowledge engineering. He has also been involved in giving Iliad National Library of Medicine workshops.

Michael Lincoln, M.D., and Charles Turner, Ph.D., have played major roles in implementing and evaluating Iliad in the University of Utah Medical School curriculum.

Joseph G. Lambert, M.D., and G. Eric Morgan, L.P.N., championed the concept of "display logic" and ideas about data drivers. Along with Katherine Sward, R.N., and Suzanne Miller, R.N., they have extensively tested the Iliad medical expert system and offered numerous suggestions for improvements.

Many clinicians have served as expert consultants for the development of the Iliad knowledge base, including for cardiology, Bruce Bray, M.D.; vascular, Clynn Ford, M.D.; endocrine and metabolism, Frank Tyler, M.D.; gastrointestinal enterology, David Bjorkman, M.D.; hematology, Stan Altman, M.D.; pulmonary medicine, Attilio Renzetti, M.D.; infectious disease, Larry Reimer, M.D.; nephrology, Martin Gregory, M.D.; rheumatology, Jim Williams, M.D.; neurology, John Roberts, M.D., Chris Jones, M.D., Greg Call, M.D., and John Adair, M.D.; psychiatry/mental health, Nate Currier, M.D. and Cathryn Tessnow, M.S.W.; dermatology, David Hansen, M.D. and Marta Petersen, M.D.; OB/GYN, Marsh Poulson,

M.D.; pediatrics, Paul Wirkus, M.D. and Richard Waldmann, M.D.; ophthalmology, Thomas Clinch, M.D.; and sports medicine, Alan Newman, M.D.

We thank Nina Dougherty and Mary Youngkin for supporting the knowledge engineering efforts with relevant literature references.

Many generous physicians and patients, too numerous to list here, have contributed images to the Iliad digitized image library.

Eric Lepage, M.D., translated Iliad into French; Peter Huber, M.D., translated Iliad into German; Alvaro Margolis, M.D., M.S., translated Iliad into Spanish; and INS Japan is translating Iliad into Japanese.

This book could not have been written without the simultaneous development of the Iliad application and Iliad Knowledge Engineering Tools by the staff of the Medical Informatics Department and Applied Medical Informatics. Major contributors to the development of the Iliad application are Chinli Fan, M.S., Robb Cundick, Ph.D., QiKang Sun, M.S., Alan Goates, Loren Erickson, and Wenshao Wang, M.S. Major contributors to the development of the Iliad KE tools are Kent Ward, M.S., QiKang Sun, M.S., Chinli Fan, M.S., and Robb Cundick, Ph.D.

Contents

1
Background and Legacy

Overview

The field of medical expert systems was reviewed by Reggia and Tuhrim in 1985,[1] by P. Miller in 1988,[2] and by R. Miller in 1994.[3] Most of their observations, which are still true today, are summarized here.

Why Build Medical Expert Systems?

The "information explosion" in recent decades has made it impossible for practicing physicians (even specialists) to keep up with all the information that would be potentially useful in making optimal clinical judgments. As a result, it is not suprising that empirical studies have demonstrated that physicians do not always make optimal decisions. Computer-assisted medical decision-making systems (also called medical expert systems) are intended to support (not replace) physicians and other health care providers, by "complementing their natural ability to make judgments with the computer's memory, reliability and processing capabilities." Other motivations for building medical expert systems include potential educational value and use as intelligent interfaces to clinical databases.[1]

Definitions

For developing medical expert systems, the input is typically a description of some specific patient (i.e., age, sex, risk factors, symptoms, signs, lab data) and the output is useful summative information about that person (e.g., diagnosis, treatment suggestions). A medical expert system contains at least two basic components: a **knowledge base** (KB) and an **inference mechanism**. The KB is a collection of encoded knowledge required to solve problems in some medical area. The inference mechanism (or inference engine) is a computer program that, given a case description, uses the information in the KB to generate new information about the case.

Individuals who use a medical expert system to assist them with a problem are **users**. Expert physicians who provide information for development of the KB are called **medical experts**. Those who design and develop the supporting software are referred to as **knowledge engineers**.

General Design Questions and Related Issues

In designing medical expert systems, there are some general fundamental problems. First, **knowledge acquisition**: how do we translate human knowlege as it currently exists in medical textbooks, journal articles, clinical databases, and the minds of physicians into abstract representations in a computer? Second, **knowledge representation**: how do we represent human knowledge in terms of data structures that can be processed by a computer? Third, **inference generation**: how do we use these abstract data structures to generate useful information in the context of a specific case?

Related issues include these:

How to determine the best representation for any given problem?
How to design software tools to facilitate system building and management?
How to manipulate the knowledge to provide explanations to the user?
How to verify and update the knowledge base?
How to evaluate and validate medical expert systems?

State of the Art

In spite of 25 years of research and testing, medical expert systems have had little impact on the day-to-day decision making of physicians and other health care professionals (except for some small systems noted below).

Several problems limiting the development and use of such expert systems are responsible for the lack of impact, e.g., as follow:

Existing medical expert systems are far from being completely accurate and reliable.
The development of medical expert system is costly in both time and money.
There is significant "physician resistance" to using medical expert systems. This is partly because physicians have not been convinced that such systems are useful and cost effective. Other reasons include a natural resistance to change, general computer ignorance, and lack of time necessary to interact with the computer.
There is a general lack of large, reliable clinical databases (especially those containing signs and symptoms) that could be useful in the design and use of medical expert systems.

Medicine is a complex field because of the inherent complexity of the
human body and disease processes. Consequently, there is an enormous
amount of medically relevant knowledge.

The pathophysiological processes underlying many diseases are poorly
understood.

Domains of medicine are notoriously idiosyncratic.

There is often a lack of an objective gold standard that can be used to
determine truth.

There is tremendous latitude in practice variation and subjective judgment.

It is apparent, at least to those working in the field, that all these problems are solvable. Also, there are encouraging trends:

Growing availability, improved performance, and falling cost of hardware

Growing availability, improved performance, and falling cost of software

Improved cost-effectiveness of building systems (resulting from decreased
cost of hardware, better software tools, and more knowledgeable system
architects)

Continuing work on basic science research in medicine, computer science,
and medical informatics

Increased computerization of patient data and availability of clinical databases

Continuing assessment of systems in clinical settings

Improved attitudes toward and familiarity with computers on the part of
health care professionals

Health care reform, which is imposing financial and quality of care constraints on providers that favor the development of an electronic medical
record and computerized systems for implementation of practice guidelines and automated outcomes research

The development of standards to ease the exchange of information between
systems (e.g., HL7,[4] Arden syntax,[5])

A number of small, focused medical decision support systems are widely
used, e.g., ECG interpretation,[6] automated differential blood count ana-
lyzers,[7] and blood gas and pulmonary function test interpretation.[3]

Knowledge Representation and Computation Methodologies

Medical decision support systems have been categorized in a number of
ways: clinical algorithms, clinical databanks that include analytic functions,
mathematical pathophysiologic models, pattern recognition systems, Bayesian statistical systems, decision analytical systems, and symbolic reasoning
or expert systems.[8]

Real-world diagnostic systems involve a constant balancing of theory
(model complexity) and practicality (ability to construct and maintain adequate medical knowledge bases, and ability to create systems that respond

to users' needs in acceptably short time intervals). Systems should take into account gradations of symptoms, the degree of uncertainty in patients and physicians/users regarding a finding, the severity of each illness under consideration, the pathophysiologic mechanisms of disease, and the time course of illnesses.[3]

In medical diagnosis, it is sometimes advantageous to reason categorically (causally) and other times to reason probabilistically. Most knowledge representation and computation methodologies used in medical expert systems today can be broadly categorized as rule based, probablistic, or some combination of these. Other worthy implementations exist but are not considered here.

Rule-Based Medical Expert Systems

Medical knowledge in rule-based systems is represented as a set of conditional rules or production rules. Each rule has the basic form: *IF* antecedents *THEN* consequences.

Probably the best-known production rule system is the MYCIN system.[9] The MYCIN system was developed originally to provide consultation advice on diagnosis of and therapy for bacteremias. It provides advice to the user via the consultation program, which includes an interactive question-and-answer module. The source of domain-specific knowledge is a set of production rules, each with a premise and an action. The production rules are implemented as modular segments of code so that the KB and inference engine are integrated together. One reason for this configuration is that the system can "backward chain" to obtain an explanation for advice given to the user. The program has been extensively tested and is apparently well accepted by clinicians.

The production rule approach seems well suited for relatively small KBs as the complexity of designing, using, and maintaining such systems increases rapidly as the number of rules increase.[3] Many of the data-driven, warning, and reminder systems incorporated into medical record systems use, in effect, rules to "diagnose" conditions that trigger the reminders. Examples include the Regenstrief Clinic System (CARE) developed by McDonald et al.[10] and the HELP system developed by Warner et al.[11,12]

A second problem is that in most if not all such systems there is no weighting of the individual elements. In other words, all items are treated as if they had the same frequency of occurrence in the population. Another difficulty with rule-based systems is that expressing medical problem solving as a single set of context-independent rules is an impossible or difficult task in many cases.[1] For example, a rule-based program for localization of damage to the central nervous system was developed to evaluate MYCIN-like production system methodology.[13] "A collection of rules was found to be a poor representation for neurological localization knowledge because such information is conceptually organized in a 'frame-like fashion' and is very context-dependent."

Many frame-based/rule-based systems have been developed in recent years, e.g., the HELP system.[11,12] Frames are, in effect, tables of findings that are separate from the rules. This design is less restrictive than the strict production rule approach but still suffers from the fact that it is difficult to create rules that fit all cases (especially of a disease presentation).

Probabilistic Medical Expert Systems

Bayesian classification has long been a major approach used to construct medical expert systems. Such systems represent knowledge as a set of probabilities, prior probabilities of outcomes, and conditional probabilities of input features. The inference mechanism applies Bayes' theory to this information to calculate the probability of each possible outcome when given a description of a particular case. The assumption is often made in practice that the individual symptoms are independent. If this assumption is used, the KB does not require the potentially astronomically large set of 2^n joint probabilities for each disease, where n is the total number of findings in all the diseases.

There are numerous examples of Bayesian medical expert systems, e.g., for the diagnosis of the cause of acute abdominal pain,[14] diagnosis of congenital heart disease,[15] classification of stroke,[16] diagnosis of solitary pulmonary nodules,[17] and diagnosis of thyroid disorders.[18] In each case, these workers reported that a computer program based on this model performed at a level approaching that of an expert in the respective field.

Certain criticisms have been made regarding Bayesian classification. First, Bayesian classification typically requires one to assume (falsely) that a patient's signs and symptoms are independent (and sometimes that the set of diseases is mutually exclusive), an assumption that can result in loss of performance. Second, the suggestion has often been made that Bayesian medical expert systems will not be usable at a location other than that where the original data were collected. Third, the difficulty in obtaining all the necessary probabilities may be prohibitive. Because these probabilities are usually not available, they must either be measured or estimated. Obtaining actual data is a time-consuming alternative that is often not possible because of cost. On the other hand, subjective estimation of probabilities by physicians and others has repeatedly been shown to be unsatisfactory.[1]

The original Bayesian models collected all the data for a case before performing the calculation. Gorry and Barnett were probably the first to suggest the use of sequential Bayes.[19] Their system operated in an interactive mode. The user of the program engaged in a dialogue with the program, entering data as they became available. After each piece of data was entered, the program would recalculate its probabilites and inform the user of its new results.

Lichtenstein[20] studied the effect of nonindependence in Bayesian classi-fication. He concluded that Bayesian systems are "robust with respect to the conditional independence assumption" and maintained that developers of such systems need only correct for severe violations. This was found to be particularly true in the so-called multimembership classification model in which the existence of each disorder is considered separately.[21]

Bayesian expert systems use various strategies to minimize violations of conditional independence. The most common approach is to "cluster" con-ditionally dependent features into a complex of features and to estimate the multivariate conditional distribution of this complex. Ben-Bassat et al.[21] developed a sequential multimembership classification model in which they introduced an additional strategy for resolving dependencies. Highly de-pendent features within a given disorder pattern are "marked." Once one of them is observed, the probability of diseases that use it is revised. When other features that correlate with that finding are observed, the disease probabilities are not revised. This approach partially prevented falsely com-pounding the effect of the nonindependent findings (however, it did not take into account the fact that the first finding might not be the most important item in the cluster).

These workers also showed that the Bayesian model tolerates large deviations in the a priori (i.e., the frequency of the disease in the pertinent population) and conditional probabilities (the true positive and false posi-tive frequencies). The a priori and the likelihood ratio (i.e., true positive/false positive) may deviate within a range of 65% to 135% and still produce posterior probabilities (see Chapter 3) that vary by 10% or less. Other strengths of their system included an online, multiuser environment, the ability to use negative as well as positive information, and the use of hierarchical relationships among diseases.

Bayesian networks (also called belief networks)[22-25] provide a method for formally representing probabilistic dependencies and independence. Belief networks consist of a directed, acyclic graph containing nodes whose link strengths are represented by probabilities. Relationships among observa-tions, intermediate states, and diagnoses can be expressed on a continuum from full independence to full causal dependency. In comparison with sequential Bayesian representations, belief networks require numerous additional probabilities and much more computer processing power for a given system.

Hierarchical Knowledge

Reggia reported, while developing his expert system for neurological local-ization, that it was convenient to organize the KB using a "natural inference hierarchy." Successively higher levels in the hierarchy represented greater levels of abstraction of the information about the patient.[13]

Similarly, Kulikowski made use of a natural disease hierarchy in the development of the CASNET/Glaucoma consultation system.[26] In describing the construction of the knowledge base, he noted that "a descriptive scheme for modeling diseases can be conceived as a structure that contains observations and concepts layered in increasing order of abstraction and complexity." This system is essentially composed of nested decision frames, which he refers to as decision nodes. The lowest level of abstraction contains direct observations (i.e., signs, symptoms, and test results). The second plane of nodes contains "anatomical-physiological states, which serve as summaries of pathological conditions that can be linked together by cause and effect and other semantic relations to describe the dynamic process of disease evolution. These states are often not directly observable or measurable entities, but must be inferred from the specific observations made at level one." Examples of his pathophysiological clusters are "increased intraocular pressure," "cupping of the optic disc," and "visual field loss."

Kulakowski describes disease mechanisms by causal pathways. Various classification structures are imposed on the network for the purpose of defining diagnostic, prognostic, and treatment categories. This approach is powerful but is limited by the fact that each pathophysiological state is restricted to only three values, i.e., confirmed, denied, or undetermined. Based on these values, therapies can be ranked by indices of severity and effectiveness.

Hybrid Models and Ambitious Adaptations

INTERNIST-1[27] was the first medical expert system to assume the ambitious task of diagnosing all diseases in internal medicine. INTERNIST-1 and its successor QMR (Quick Medical Reference)[28,29] make use of frame-based disease profiles that comprise its KB. Each frame lists findings that can occur in patients with each disease.

Two clinical variables are associated with each manifestation in a disease profile: an evoking strength and a frequency. The evoking strength answers the question; "given a finding, how strongly should I consider this diagnosis to be the explanation." The frequency is an estimate of how often patients with the disease have the finding (i.e., the sensitivity). In addition, each manifestation is assigned a disease-independent import score. The import score is the global importance of the finding—that is, "the extent to which one is compelled to explain its presence in any patient."

The evoking strength, frequency, and import are expressed on a scale of 0 to 5. These numbers are summed for each frame in a given case. By "inverting" the disease profiles, an exhaustive differential diagnostic list for each finding is obtained by the computer. These lists are then used to construct a grand differential diagnostic list corresponding to a patient's findings.

A similar approach was taken by the developers of the DXplain system.[30,31] DXplain is a medical expert system that generates a differential diagnosis from a given list of clinical manifestations. Its KB includes several thousand diseases and about twice as many clinical terms including demographics, symptoms, signs, and laboratory findings. Each term has two disease-dependent attributes, Term Frequency and Evoking Strength, and a disease-independent Term Importance. Term frequency is a measure of how frequent the finding occurs in a particular disease. The evoking strength indicates how strongly one should think of a particular disease, given the presence of the finding.

In 1988, the Iliad medical expert system was first reported.[32-34] This system also proposed to cover all of internal medicine as well as some specialties. The model for this expert system made use of some previously developed ideas and some unique additions. The KB was composed of frame-based disease descriptions related to each other in such a way that any frame could use any other frame as a complex finding if it made sense medically. The inference engine was sequential Bayes. Nonindependence was handled through the use of clusters and "or groups."

The presumed unique features of Iliad included the following:

A combination of Bayesian and Boolean (i.e., rule-based) frames
A hierarchical data dictionary (of all constituent findings) that makes use of inferencing
The use of "Or groups" in which nonindependent findings in a Bayesian frame only allow the strongest known finding in the group to be used in the calculation
A best information algorithm (that made suggestions on what to do next), which was based both on information content and the cost of getting the information.

In 1989, the concept of passing partial information between frames was introduced[35] in Iliad. This idea was not new in itself, but the use of the "closeness" concept was. The closeness concept facilitated passing of partial information between Bayesian and Boolean frames and also allowed frames to have both positive and negative information simultaneously. A "minimal diagnosis" algorithm was also added, which allowed the user to select from a set of competing diagnoses the one that best explained the patient's findings at any given time. In 1990, so-called data relations and word relations were added to Iliad to make use of nonexplicit information in the dictionary.[36] These additions built on work being done with the Unified Medical Language System (UMLS) project.[37]

Almost all the top-level (i.e., final diagnosis) frames in Iliad are Bayesian. There are several reasons for this. First, the a priori probability sets the starting point of each disease, so that common diseases start out being much more likely than rare diseases. Second, a definitive rule will not always apply in the early stages of the workup before obtaining specific data; there will always be variability in the way patients present. Third, Boolean frames force the user to exclude potentially useful information. For example, some disorders described in DSM-IV (Diagnostic & Statistical Manual of Mental Disorders)[38] require that no organic disorder be present. A Boolean frame would have to exclude the possibility of diagnosing a psychiatric disorder in a patient with a concomitant unrelated organic disorder. As previously noted, in Boolean frames constituent items are generally weighted in a very crude way, i.e., by the way the items are related in the logic. In an Iliad Bayesian frame, each item can be specifically "tuned." Theoretically, it is possible to assign intrinsic weights to items used in Boolean frames by using a data dictionary tied to a particular patient population (see Chapter 3), but this is not being done in current systems.

Iliad and QMR both have the limitation of being stand-alone systems (in contradistinction to DXplain). Hopefully, client/server versions or Internet versions will be available in the near future. A more serious limitation at the moment is the lack of integration with a patient database. Another serious limitation is the inability to explicitly handle time.

In terms of performance (accuracy, completeness, etc.), both systems have been tested by others with less than stellar results. However, these results can probably be taken with a grain of salt because the studies were done with outdated versions of the expert system applications and because the users were not trained in the use of the systems. Also, because of the enormous size of the KBs, an enormous amount of testing is required to reach an optimum performance level. That level likely has not been reached for either system.

QMR has an advantage over Iliad in that it is able to form diagnoses in specific problem areas. On the other hand, both QMR and DXplain use semiquantitative scoring algorithms and do not make explicit use of nesting or intermediate complex findings.

One limitation of Iliad (and probably QMR and DXplain as well) is the handling of negative information. The basic problem is that there are frequently several competing diseases on the diagnostic differential list for a given patient. As more data are collected, one of these diseases will become more likely than the others. This fact should somehow make the other diseases less likely at the same time. Iliad handles this problem by adding significant negative findings to individual disease descriptions. This approach is sometimes cumbersome and not entirely effective. A more global solution would be desirable.

An additional Iliad innovation (concurrent with this publication) is the Iliad KE tool (see Chapter 9 and Appendix 3). Other systems have KE tools, but the Iliad KE tool is a stand-alone application (included with this book) that can be used for teaching purposes and to design one's own expert system. The use of this tool will allow testing of many general knowledge engineering concepts independent of the Iliad expert system.

2
The Expert System Model

Introduction to Modeling

Medical informatics is the branch of science concerned with the use of computers and communication technology to acquire, store, analyze, communicate, and display medical information and knowledge to facilitate understanding and improve the accuracy, timeliness, and reliability of decision making.[39] Understanding an observation is defined as the recognition of the relationship between what is observed and some prior observations or communication. A generalization that describes the relationships among such a set of observations is called a **model** of the set of observations or system. Decision making frequently involves the use of models. The subject matter in this volume is designed to assist the reader in learning to build a model of a system and implement the model using a computer so as to perform some useful intellectual task. Medical diagnosis is used as the principal example.

Building a model of a system is an everyday experience for each of us. By making a drawing of an object or taking a photograph of it, one has built a model of the object that can be used to convey understanding. Even more commonly, we communicate an observation to another person using words. These spoken or written words are a model representing the observer's interpretation of the object being observed. The words are chosen by the observer, who is the model builder, to represent the specific features of the object or experience he or she wishes to convey. A model is always just an approximation of the real object or experience. The choice of which features to include in a model and which to ignore becomes the key to the model's usefulness.

We create models to map complex phenomena into the realm of human understanding. Models are always simplified descriptions of their real-world counterparts. For an observation to be useful, it must first be put in some context that is familiar to the observer. In other words, it must be associated with a model, either implied or explicit, in the mind of the observer. Models represent our perception of how things fit together. Models can be viewed as a means for representing theories and hypotheses to be tested. Models can also be used to predict subsequent events and provide a basis for experimental design. When experimental results fail to conform to predictions by the model, new understanding is reached, and a new or revised model must be developed. Thus, models provide an important foundation for the scientific method itself.

A model is judged by its ability to describe those relationships in a system that account for the important features of its behavior in the most simple and understandable way and which use attributes of the system that can be conveniently observed or measured and are familiar to those who will use it. A model provides a basis for understanding and explaining a system.

The danger of making models, of course, is that they may be wrong (in whole or in part) and that they may be oversimplified. Consequently, models need to be validated. Otherwise, they may do more damage than good because, if they are wrong, they can deceive the naive user into accepting them as reality. The more a model explains and the more predictive it is (i.e., consistent with experiment), the more confidence we have in it.

An **expert system** is a special kind of model. It is a model of a decision process. It is an attempt to represent, in an approximate form that is executable by a computer, the logical processes employed by an expert in a particular subject area to decide among two or more alternative conclusions. Such system can be useful as a consultant, as a standard for critiquing observed behavior, for classification of specific observations, for prompting and alerting based on prediction of future outcomes, and as an aid to learning.

An expert system is a model capable of performing tasks that would be considered intelligent if performed by a human. Indeed, these systems have two basic components that distinguish them from other computer models. The first component is a **knowledge base** that contains the specific elements which constitute a given field of expertise, usually represented as a set of tables or lists and rules for drawing conclusions from observations. The second component of an expert system is called the **inference engine**. This component is mainly independent of the content of the knowledge base; it is the computer program capable of accepting observations and using the knowledge base to draw conclusions and make suggestions as to how to proceed in solving an instance of a problem in the domain of its knowledge.

Building an expert system model in a given problem area requires formal definitions and structures for all elements of the model. These elements include the observations, the logical relationships, the inferencing mechanisms, the interfaces to the user and other sources of information, and the specification of who will provide input and receive output from the model. Building and testing each of these elements (i.e., **knowledge engineering**) requires a team consisting of at least one expert in performing the intellectual task to be modeled and one or more knowledge engineers who understand the knowledge engineering process. This book is designed as a tool to guide and train the knowledge engineer.

In the case of a medical diagnostic expert system, pathological processes are modeled as decision "frames" by selecting, weighting, and associating findings (i.e., patient data such as symptoms, physical exam manifestations, and laboratory results) that are thought to be caused by a particular disease.

Choosing a System to Model

In choosing an intellectual task to model with the help of a computer, one must clearly define the role of the expert system in performing that task for a user. The task should be one that is performed repeatedly, that would likely be performed by someone other than the expert, and that requires a significant intellectual effort or access to knowledge not easily available to the user.

Medical diagnosis has been the favorite area for development of expert systems in medicine for several reasons. Examination of these reasons will provide some insight into what features to look for in selecting an area to model as an expert system.

The representation of the subject "diagnosis" in printed form is difficult to use as an aid when confronted with a patient with a puzzling set of symptoms. If a book or other form of publication is organized by disease, one cannot usually access the diagnosis by looking for a symptom or finding or a set of findings. The literature is not indexed by symptoms, physical findings, or test results, as is evident by the scarcity of such terms in the MeSH (Medical Subject Heading) vocabulary used for indexing. Even if a book is organized by disease manifestations, combinations of findings are hard to interpret.

There are various stages at which many diseases might be recognized or at least suspected, and there are many tests that might be performed to confirm the diagnosis. Thus, it is a challenge to form an appropriate differential diagnosis early in the diagnostic workup to direct the selection of tests that will establish the diagnosis in the most cost-effective way.

Much of the intellectual challenge in medicine is in the broad area of diagnosis. However, after the initial diagnosis is established and under treatment, the patient must be monitored for complications, deterioration caused by the disease, and adverse effects of the treatment itself. Each of these activities can also be modeled as a decision-making or pattern recognition process.

Treatment protocols or critical pathways for patient management can be followed using paper forms. However, a computer-based expert system representation of these algorithms does offer the ability to prompt the user and collect the data documenting the process for later analysis of variations from the prescribed standard.

Before starting the construction of a medical expert system, one should determine how, where, and by whom the system would be used in the patient care process. Will it function as a consulting, a critiquing, or a learning tool? Will it be used in a stand-alone mode or will it be interfaced to a database? Will the users be physicians, other professionals, or lay people including the patients themselves? Will the interaction between the user and the system be at a single point in time or will it involve a sequence of encounters? The answer to each of these questions will influence not only the selection of modeling tools but also the choice of terms used to represent patient findings or observations and how the time course of events is expressed.

Is the domain of the knowledge base sufficient to cover all relevant decision alternatives? For example, the domain may involve only the diagnosis of problems encountered in pregnant women presenting in the emergency department with vaginal bleeding. Such a narrow domain of knowledge is only useful in a setting where the criteria for patient selection are carefully observed.

Is sufficient knowledge available in the subject area of interest and in what form does that knowledge currently exist? Do you have one or more experts on the subject who are willing to work with you? Do you have an environment available to test the performance of the system before putting it to use? Because an expert system should perform like an expert or should help the nonexpert perform like an expert, choosing the right expert(s) to help build the system is a vital step in the the knowledge engineering process.

The user interface to the expert system can facilitate or restrict the use of the system, no matter how good the knowledge base. Ideally, this interface should also be tailored to the user and the environment. If this cannot be done because of lack of access to the source code, selection of the system to model must also be influenced by the available user interface. Multiple confusing poorly designed screens will limit use of the system, no matter how good it is.

How detailed should the representation be? The amount of detail (level of sophistication) of the diagnostic frames will be determined by a number of factors, including the following:

The proficiency and knowledge of potential users
The availability of diagnostic information
The availability of numerical data
How well the pathogenesis of constituent diseases is understood
How complicated a disease is
How much variability there is in disease presentation
How much detail the data acquisition process can accommodate.

Choosing a Model

Patient management protocols can be represented using a simple branching model in which the branching at each node is dependent only on past or existing data values. No attempt is made in building the decision model to express the likely costs or benefits explicitly, and no attempt is made to incorporate uncertainty in the form of probabilities into the model.[9]

A more sophisticated model makes use of decision analysis.[40,41] In the formal decision analysis model, the decision process is represented as a branching tree structure where each branch is labeled as either a decision node or an outcome node. Each outcome associated with a node is labeled with a probability, and the sum of all the probabilities from such a node must equal 1. Each terminal branch of the decision tree has a cost and/or a benefit associated with it. Mathematical expressions can be used to represent both probabilities and outcomes to make these parameters dependent on patient-specific values (e.g., life expectancy is a function of the patient's age). Computer applications are available to construct such models and are used in some places to calculate which pathway (series of decisions) through the decision tree will result in the best outcome for the patient. This approach allows a user to choose among the decisions at the base of the tree knowing that it is the one most likely to be best for the patient. The decision analysis model is used when a series of action-oriented decisions must be made, probability estimates of outcome from each action are known, and it is possible to estimate the outcome costs and benefits in common terms (monetary, "good days of life," etc.).

The most common decision model is "rule based," i.e., involving logical operators (i.e., the Boolean model). Rules are expressed as "if (condition) is true, then (action)," where "condition" may be any set of previously defined variables separated by logical operators with or without numerical operators [e.g., (i) True if a or b or (c and d); (ii) True if a >37C and 2 of (b,c,d)]. A Boolean model may be the appropriate choice in cases where the knowledge already exists as a set of rules or definitions. A good example of this is a system for interpretation of electrocardiographic (ECG) waveforms.[42] Empirical knowledge has accumulated over many years establishing definitions such as the criteria for left bundle branch block. Clinicians have learned to correlate these interpretations with diagnoses and prognoses in a useful way, and most commercial ECG machines now include interpretation rules.

In other circumstances the criteria for diagnosis may be established as a set of rules by a clinical organization such as the American College of Rheumatology.[43] Care must be taken, however, that the use for which the rules were defined matches the needs of the environment in which the expert system will operate. For example, the rules established for diagnosing disseminated lupus erythematosis in this study were criteria for including patients in a large-scale clinical trial. These rules did not work well in the

Iliad expert system when used to diagnose patients early in the course of their disease. In this case, a probabilistic model proved to be more useful. The same was true for multiple myeloma and numerous psychiatric diseases (defined as rules in DSM-IV).[38]

The task of recognizing the cause of a patient's complaints by establishing a diagnosis usually involves uncertainty. Definitive tests are often expensive and sometimes even risky for the patient. Thus, it is important that an ordered list of diagnostic possibilites be established early in the workup that may be used as hypotheses to be tested. Most successful diagnostic systems incorporate probability estimates or some other weighting algorithm to establish such a list. These pattern recognition approaches can use any number of findings in combination to provide a measure of certainty of a set of diagnoses or intermediate decisions. If there is an independent "gold standard" by which to determine the accuracy of a decision, then a probabilistic representation is more appropriate. It is inherently more flexible and can accommodate parameters used by experts such as prevalence of the disease.

Because the manifestations of a disease often vary as the disease progresses or as a result of therapeutic interventions, time becomes an important variable to take into account in building a diagnostic model. Time can be incorporated to some extent into the disease descriptions using such phrases as "occurring within the last week" or "lasting for >1 month." For use as a diagnostic aid in a clinical setting, however, it is desirable to link the expert system to a patient database in which data from multiple visits can be entered into the system and time between visits or during a single visit can be formally incorporated into the disease descriptions. Such a new dimension places additional requirements on the model and the database to which it is linked.[12,44,45] Concepts must be expressed in both the patient database and the expert system using similar data structures or a system for translation must be developed.[46]

Expert systems are of little use once the sine qua non data are available. Expert systems are most useful during the early and intermediate stages of the patient workup. A diagnostic expert system should suggest hypotheses to consider and appropriate tests to perform to better refine the differential diagnosis. The sequence of appearance of disease manifestations often differs from patient to patient. Because it is often difficult or impossible to define rules to cover all the variations in the presentation pattern, probabilistic models may be more appropriate for many diseases.

Many areas of medicine are amenable to a pattern recognition approach to decision making in which a number of findings in combination will adjust the certainties of various final outcomes or intermediate decisions. If an intermediate decision to be made (in the diagnostic process) is by definition (e.g., a rule defined by a clinical organization), then a rule-based representation is appropriate. If there is an independent "gold standard" by which to determine the accuracy of a decision, then a probabilistic representation is more appropriate because it is inherently more flexible and more powerful. A key difference is that, in the probabilistic case, each item has one or more probabilities associated with it which can be independently adjusted.

Choosing a model will depend on the nature of the observation data. Observations may be binary (present or absent) or continuous (e.g., age, WBC). Continuous data can be converted to binary (age >20 years) before or after entering it into the expert system. If the conversion is done by the system, each decision can have its own threshold, and multiple thresholds can be used within a given decision process. Information is lost each time a continuous value is converted to a binary representation. The creator of an expert system must make many such decisions about simplicity of use and sophistication of the expert system. In this regard, when discrete intervals are used, the number of intervals will be determined by clinical relevance, availability of reliable and pertinent data, and ultimate effect on performance of the system. Certain calculated data, such as "expected total cholesterol levels for females of various ages," are naturally represented as a continuous function. This imposes yet another requirement on the model.

If two diseases have nearly identical presentations, it may not make sense to include them as separate entities in the system. Likewise, if two diseases can only be differentiated on the basis of a bacterial culture or a histological exam, it may not be desirable to separate them, especially if the treatments are the same.

Medical knowledge varies by domain for a number of reasons, e.g., dermatology is a very descriptive specialty, cardiology relies heavily on patient history data, gastroenterology and endocrinology rely heavily on laboratory data, and pulmonary medicine relies heavily on radiological evidence. Some specialties have come into being fairly recently, while others have decades of clinical information upon which to draw. Consequently, building a large medical expert system covering multiple domains may require a combination of different models or different variations of a model. How information and uncertainty is passed between submodels must be consistently carried out and defined explicitly if possible.

3
Iliad: The Model Used for This Text

The Frame Concept

Building Individual Decision Frames

In the case of a diagnostic expert system, each disease or diagnostic decision can be represented as a list or table called a frame. The decision frame contains the relevant findings (i.e., disease manifestations), associated logic, and probabilities in the case of a probabilistic (e.g., Bayesian) frame. Frames can be represented in different ways, e.g., Bayesian, Boolean, and value-type Boolean frames are used in the Iliad expert system.

Bayesian Frames

Bayesian frames represent decisions/diseases by making use of a priori, true positive (TP), and false positive (FP) probability estimates, as shown in this example:

Industrial bronchitis (a priori = .0014)

		TP	FP
a.	•At risk for industrial bronchitis	.99	.001
b.	•Chronic cough with mucoid sputum	.99	.01
c.	•Airways obstruction by spirometry	.25	.02

Note: The "•" indicates a complex finding defined in another frame.

The a priori is the fraction of patients in the disease population with a given disease (patients can have multiple diseases). The TP is the fraction of patients having a given finding in a given disease. The FP is the fraction of patients in the disease population who have a given finding but do not have the given disease. The value of the frame is determined by sequentially using the Bayes equation (see following) for each finding for which information is available to adjust the posteriori probability. The first calculation uses the a priori as the prior probability (i.e., the initial probability of the disease). Subsequent calculations use the previous posteriori probability as a revised prior probability. Because the Bayes equation assumes that the items in the frame are independent, it is necessary to have some means of formally enforcing this constraint; failure to do so will result in overconfidence of the system. Two methods used in Iliad are described next, i.e., the use of the "or" construct and the use of clusters.

Empirically, it can be shown that a "small" amount of nonindependence generally has little effect on the final calculation. In practice, it is usually not possible to completely avoid some nonindependence among findings in a Bayesian frame. Theoretically, the actual amount of nonindependence could be taken into account if the data were available (i.e., "Bayesian networks"). The system can also be "tuned," by adjusting the sensitivities and specificities to compensate for overconfidence resulting from nonindependence.

Experience with Iliad development suggests that other uncertainties are frequently more important than nonindependence, e.g., those associated with the actual estimates of a prioris, sensitivities, and specificities, lack of understanding of disease etiologies, differences in presentation in different patients because of genotypic differences and multiple concurrent diseases, and disagreements among experts and knowledge engineers as to how the disease frame should be modeled.

Boolean Frames

Boolean frames are simply a list of findings with an associated rule that determines the value of the frame based on the presence or absence of various findings in the list, e.g.:

Infarction chest pain
   a. Hx of chest pain at rest
   b. Hx of chest pain next to or under patient's breastbone (sternum)
   c. Hx of chest pain that seems to squeeze or constrict (crushing)
   d. Hx of chest pain radiating to the shoulder, arm, or neck
   e. Hx of chest pain relieved by rest, completely
   f. Hx of chest pain relieved by nitroglycerin, completely
   g. •Pleuritic chest pain
   h. •Chest wall pain
True if a and b and (c or d) and not (e or f or g or h).

For every "True if" statement, there is an inherent "False if" statement that can be generated by replacing all "or"s with "and"s, all "and"s with "or"s, then preceding each finding with a "not" if one is not present or removing a "not" if it is present, e.g., True if (a or b) and not c → False if (not a and not b) or c.

Theoretically, certainty weights could be included in the logic. An elegant method was attempted in the Iliad expert system using frequencies of disease findings stored in the data dictionary (see Chapter 4). The basic idea is straightforward: if the total frequency of every finding is known in the population, then the importance of a given finding in a Boolean frame will be inversely proportional to this frequency. In other words, rare findings, when they are present, are more important than common ones. Weighting factors can be calculated by dividing each finding in a frame by its frequency multiplied by some normalizing factor that adds all the weights to 1. This approach was eventually abandoned in Iliad because (i) not all the frequencies were known accurately; (ii) it was not clear what frequencies to assign to complex findings (i.e., findings which were themselves subframes); and (iii) when findings were negative, the weights did not seem to work as expected. However, for smaller systems, such an approach may be feasible and more appropriate.

In general, Boolean frames are less powerful than Bayesian frames because there are fewer numbers to adjust, especially if there are no weighting factors. It is difficult, in practice, to come up with a rule that is true for all patients in all cases, e.g., chest pain patterns. On the other hand, Boolean frames are simpler to generate and maintain and usually easier to understand by users. In addition, they are a convenient way of grouping nonindependent items, they may be used to represent a concept such as a pathological process, and they are easier to process by the inference engine.

Value Frames

Value frames are a type of Boolean frame that do not allow the passage of partial information (see following). In other words, they are not assigned a value until enough information is available to come to some final decision. There are two types of value frames. Type I returns a true or false, and type II value frames perform a calculation and return a numerical value.

Nested Frames: Clusters

Each diagnostic frame can include complex findings that are themselves composed of subframes or "clusters" (i.e., a set of similar or interdependent

findings/observations) of related findings. The term "cluster" is most appropriate when applied to pathophysiological entities, such as "dependent
edema," "lung consolidation," or "pulmonary venous congestion," which
are then subcomponents of higher level decision frames. This approach
allows management of dependent elements, which is arguably analogous to
the reasoning process of experts who tend to use "chunks" of information
in arriving at hypotheses to be tested.[47]

The Probabilistic Model: Dealing with Uncertainty

The Bayes Equation

The Bayes equation, in its simplest form, is the initial probability of the
disease multiplied by the ratio of the probability of the finding in that
disease compared to the total probability of the finding in the population of
interest:

$$P_{d/f} = P_d * \left(P_{f/d} / P_f \right)$$

where $P_{d/f}$ is the posteriori probability (i.e., the revised probability after the
finding becomes known), P_d is the a priori, $P_{f/d}$ is the sensitivity of the finding
in a disease (i.e., the true positive rate), and P_f is the probability (i.e., the
frequency) of the finding in the population. In sequential Bayes, when
subsequent findings become known, the a priori is replaced by the previous
posteriori probability. The order of the findings makes no difference in the
final outcome.

As noted, use of sequential Bayes assumes independence of findings.
Otherwise, the posteriori probability will be inappropriately high (i.e.,
overconfident) because some findings will be counted more than once.
The Bayes equation can be used to test for nonindependence because
if two findings (f1 and f2) are independent, then $P_{d/f1 \text{ then } f2}$ should equal
$P_{d/f1} \times P_{d/f2}$.

Ways of Handling the Assumption of Independence

Nonindependence can be formally handled through the use of the "or"
construct or by using constituent Boolean clusters. In the "Iron deficiency
anemia" frame (see following), "Iron deficiency," "At risk for iron deficiency," and "Chronic blood loss" are Boolean frames that include a number of nonindependent findings. The elements of an "or group" are treated
by the inference engine in a "one or the other; whichever is stronger"
manner. The importance (i.e., information content) of each finding can be
compared by calculating the true positive (TP)/false positive (FP) ratios:

.9999/.01 = 99.99, .95/.25 = 3.96, and .95/.10 = 9.5 (negative ratios are calculated as the ratios of the complements in the opposite direction). If at some point in the workup it is known that the patient has "Chronic blood loss," the ratio of 9.5 is used. If later it turns out that the patient has "Iron deficiency," then the 9.5 calculation is uncalculated and replaced with a 99.99 calculation. The ratios are not actually used in the calculation; TP and FP are used in the Bayes equation.

Iron deficiency anemia (a priori = .075)

a.	•Anemia	.999	.10
b.	•Hypochromic and microcytic RBCs	.85	.07
c.	•Iron deficiency	.9999	.01
	xor		
	•At risk for iron deficiency	.95	.25
	xor		
	•Chronic blood loss	.95	.10
d.	•Absolute reticulocyte count		
	<50,000	.90	.08
	50,000–200,000	.10	.84
	≥200,000	.001	.08
e.	•Thalassemia minor	.0008	.008

It is important to note that there are at least two types of "or"s or "or groups." For example, any of the h items in "ischemic colitis" (see below) would be considered positive evidence for the disease, even if one or more of the other items were not true. If the user had entered a "No" for "Hx of peripheral vascular disease," this would correspond to a negative information of $(1 - .05)/(1 - .8) = .95/.20 = 4.75$. If the patient also had "Hx of stroke," this would have a positive information of $.10/.04 = 2.5$. The absolute value of the negative information would exceed that of the positive. However, in this case it is not desirable for the negative information to override the positive. This is also true for the other items in this "or group." In this case, it is desirable for the inference engine to allow any positive information to be used in place of a stronger negative finding. It may be noted that the items in h could be otherwise represented in a Boolean frame with logic "True if any." This was not done in this case because the positive weights of the findings vary significantly.

Findings c_1, c_2, and c_3 in "Iron deficiency anemia" (see foregoing) are related by a different kind of "or" (designated here as an xor). For an xor type of "or group," a negative value on a more specific finding (c_1) will override a positive on the less specific findings (c_2 or c_3). (Note that the subscript designates the order of the item in the "or group.") If the patient does not have "Iron deficiency," this information should override the fact that the patient is "At risk for iron deficiency" or has "Chronic blood loss."

Ischemic colitis (a priori = .0003)

a. Age >60 years	.95	.30
b. Hx of sudden onset, cramping lower abdominal pain	.70	.03
or		
Hx of abdominal pain	.70	.15
c. •Inflammatory diarrhea	.60	.015
or		
•Endoscopic evidence of colitis	.90	.02
d. •Fever	.30	.18
e. Abdominal x-ray: evidence of intramural hemorrhage and edema in the colon	.33	.02
f. Colonic biopsy shows ischemia	.95	.0001
g. Abdominal arteriography shows vascular obstruction or venous stasis	.95	.001
h. Hx of coronary artery disease	.20	.04
or		
Hx of stroke	.10	.04
or		
Systolic BP < 90	.20	.01
or		
Hx of vasculitis	.10	.001
or		
Hx of peripheral vascular disease	.80	.05
or		
Hx of abdominal radiation therapy	.20	.01

Because all levels of azotemia in "renal failure" (see following) require creatinine to be greater than 1.5 mg/dL, all patients with renal failure should have this finding. A negative for this finding would have a ratio of .95/.001 or 950 fold. Note that a negative on items a_1, a_2, or a_3 would be very weak and not be able to override any of the other findings; thus, it was necessary to include item a_4 to provide for a strong negative finding. However, if finding a_1 is present (e.g., from a very high BUN or a very low creatinine clearance), then the negative on a_4 will not be strong enough to override it.

Renal failure (a priori = .01)

a. •Severe azotemia	.30	.0001
xor		
•Moderate azotemia	.30	.001
xor		
•Mild azotemia	.40	.04
xor		
Serum creatinine >1.5 mg/dL	.999	.05
b. •Nonspecific manifestations of renal failure	.50	.01

Severe azotemia
  a. Creatinine clearance ≤10 ml/min
  b. Serum creatinine ≥10 mg/dL
  c. BUN ≥200 mg/dL
True if any

Moderate azotemia
  a. Creatinine clearance >10 and ≤20 ml/min
  b. Serum creatinine ≥3 and <10 mg/dL
  c. BUN ≥50 and <200 mg/dL
  d. Serum creatinine 2 mg/dL on two readings at least 2 weeks apart
True if any

Mild azotemia
  a. Creatinine clearance >20 and ≤80 ml/min
  b. Serum creatinine ≥1.5 and <3 mg/dL
  c. BUN ≥20 and <50 mg/dL
True if a or (b and c)

In a less obvious example, even though "Megaloblastic anemia" and "Macrocytic anemia" are very strong findings in "Anemia of B_{12} deficiency" (see following), the lack of "Megaloblastic anemia" (which is determined by examining tissue from the bone marrow) should override "Macrocytic anemia" (which could result from folate deficiency). This is another good example of domain-specific knowledge being necessary for correct construction of the model.

Anemia of B12 deficiency (a priori = .0003)
  a. •Megaloblastic anemia   .999   .0003
     xor
     •Macrocytic anemia   .999   .003
  b. •Serum B_{12} <200 ng/mL   .9999   .00001
  c. •Subacute combined degeneration   .40   .0001

Megaloblastic anemia
  a. •Macrocytic anemia
  b. •Depressed erythropoietic activity
  c. Bone marrow shows megaloblasts
  d. Bone marrow shows giant metamyelocytes
  e. •Pancytopenia
  f. Multilobed polymorphonuclear leukocytes
  g. •Indirect hyperbilirubinemia
True if (a and b and c and g)
        or (c and e)
        or (a and c and f)
        or (a and d and e and f)

Macrocytic anemia
    a. •Anemia
    b. MCV = = =
    True if a and b > 102

Subacute combined degeneration (a priori = .00012)

a. Age >40 years	.95	.57
b. •Pernicious anemia	.80	.0004
c. •Myelopathy	.99	.002
or		
•Sensorimotor polyneuropathy	.20	.01
or		
•Optic neuritis	.05	.01
or		
•Dementia; slowly progressive	.30	.01
or		
•Delirium	.15	.01
g. Serum methyl malonic acid increased	.99	.0001
or		
Serum vitamin B_{12} <200 pg/mL	.90	.02

Probabilistic Information

Partial Information

When expert clinicians acquire part of the information necessary to make a diagnosis, they unconsciously attach some probability to that being the true diagnosis. When additional information becomes available, their certainty (probability) of the diagnosis changes accordingly. A diagnostic expert system must also have this capability if it is to emulate a human expert in a compelling manner. This behavior is a natural outcome of the sequential Bayes model in which the posteriori probability is recalculated as each finding is processed (using the previous posteriori probability as a revised a priori).

Boolean frames are more problematic. How does one allocate partial credit to a Boolean frame with a simple rule such as "True if a and 2 of (b or c or d) and not e," when only part of the information is available to fulfill the logic? In addition, a given frame may have some evidence toward being true and, at the same time, some evidence toward being false.

Iliad uses probabilistic and deterministic frames linked in a tangled hierarchy where any combination of Bayesian and Boolean frames is allowable (assuming that it makes sense clinically) and the number of nested subframes may theoretically go to any depth (although nesting should be minimized to avoid unnecessary complexity). These linked frames must dynamically communicate their current state to one another to determine:

1. How close each frame (hypothesis) is to being true or false, based on those features of the patient's illness available at a given stage in the diagnostic workup
2. How useful the acquisition of any particular new finding might be at each stage of the diagnostic process

The "Closeness to True/False" Concept

For Bayesian and Boolean frames to communicate with each other, some sort of common currency is necessary. The Iliad expert system uses the concept of "closeness to true" or "closeness to false" to express the certainty of a Bayesian or a Boolean frame in common units.

For Boolean frames, close_t and close_f vary between 0 and 1. They are essentially pseudoprobabilities, the calculation of which can be understood by considering a simple example. Consider a frame with logic "True if a and 2 of (b,c,d) and (e or f)" and a patient with findings a, b, and e true. Finding a represents 1/3 of the necessary information, "2 of (b,c,d)" represents 1/3 of the necessary information, and "(e or f)" represents 1/3 of the necessary information to become completely true (because there are three parts of the statement separated by "and" operators). So, for the patient in question, the value of the frame is $1/3 + .5(1/3) + 1/3 = 5/6$. The close_f is determined by writing and calculating the corresponding "False if" equation. In this case, it would be "False if not a or not 2 of (b,c,d) or (not e and not f)." When close_t becomes 1, close_f becomes 0, and vice versa.

To represent the state of a Bayesian frame using a commensurate measure (to the Boolean case) of closeness to being true or false, the a priori is considered the starting point. The close_t is the fraction of the distance the posteriori probability is from the a priori to 1 at any time during the analysis. The close_f is the fraction of the distance between the a priori and 0. In other words (with P = posteriori probability at any time; P_a = a priori):

$$\text{If } P > P_a$$
$$\text{close\_t} = (P - P_a)/(1 - P_a)$$
$$\text{close\_f} = 0, \text{ while}$$
$$\text{if } P < P_a$$
$$\text{close\_t} = 0$$
$$\text{close\_f} = (P_a - P)/P_a$$

In many clinical settings, P_a is close to 0 for most diseases, so $1 - P_a$ is approximately 1. Consequently, close_t is approximately equal to P, i.e., the posteriori probability.

Information Content

In many of the examples just noted, the forward (i.e., positive) ratio (i.e., TP/FP) and reverse ratio of the complements of TP and FP (i.e., $(1-FP)/(1-TP)$) were used as relative measures of importance (i.e., **information content**) in comparing findings in Bayesian frames. The forward ratio represents positive information content and the reverse ratio represents negative information content. The "most useful information" may vary depending on circumstance. In some cases, it may be desirable to factor cost, risk, or urgency into the calculation.

The ability to decide which item of information to acquire next is an important feature of an expert system's inference engine. For an expert system to behave like an expert in diagnosing a patient's problem and for it to provide the standard against which student performance will be judged, the criteria for this decision must reflect what experts would consider optimal performance.

Information Content of an Item in a Boolean Frame. The information content of an item in a Boolean frame is determined by how much the value of the item contributes toward making the frame closer to being either true or false. One method is as follows:

$$Inf\_t = \left(\text{close}\_t \text{ after item} - \text{close\_t before item}\right) \big/ \left(\text{close\_t before item}\right)$$

or

$$Inf\_f = \left(\text{close}\_f \text{ after item} - \text{close\_f before item}\right) \big/ \left(\text{close\_f before item}\right)$$

The information content (Inf) of the item is taken as the maximum of Inf_t and Inf_f. For example, consider a frame in which the logic is: True if (a or b) and c and not d. The corresponding negative logic is: False if (not a and not b) or not c or d. If, at some point in the workup, a is known to be false and c is known to be true, then it can be seen that (1) item a being false represents 50% of the way toward being completely false and (2) item c being true corresponds to 33% of the way toward being completely true. Therefore, close_t = .33 and close_f = .5. Now, suppose we learn that item d is not true. This changes close_t to .66, but does not affect close_f. So the information content of this new information is (1) inf_t = (.66 − .33)/.33 = 2 and (2) inf_f = (.5 − .5)/.5 = 0.

Information Content of an Item in a Bayesian Frame. To determine the information content (Inf) of an item in a Bayesian frame, first the posteriori probability (P_p) is calculated for each possible value (or range of values) for the finding using the current probability of the frame (P_c) as the a priori. The highest and lowest values of P_p are used to calculate positive (inf_t) and negative (Inf_f) as follows:

$$\text{If } P_p > P_c$$
$$\text{Inf}\_t = \left(P_p - P_c\right)/\left(1 - P_c\right)$$
$$\text{or if } P_p < P_c$$
$$\text{Inf}\_f = \left(P_c - P_p\right)/P_c$$
$$\text{If } P_p = P_c, \text{ then Inf}\_t = \text{Inf}\_f = 0$$

The information content (Inf) of the item is taken as the maximum of Inf_t and Inf_f.

Selecting the "Best Information" to Acquire Next. The definition of "best" used by Iliad is that item of information which will most influence (increase or decrease the probability of) the most likely diagnosis for the least cost. This can be expressed as

$$\text{utility of each finding} = \text{Inf} * \text{closeness}/\text{cost}^x$$

where "Inf" is the information content of the item for a given frame, closeness is the closeness to true or false, and x is an empirically determined exponent (Iliad uses a value of 1).

Passing Information Among Bayesian and Boolean Frames

Diagnostic frames can contain complex findings, and each of these findings can vary in value depending on the particular stage in the workup. In other words, a complex finding can be partially true (measured by close_true) or partially false (measured by close_false). If the complex finding is a Bayesian frame, the posterior probability of the frame is used as a multiplying factor to reduce the effect of the Bayesian calculation for the finding in the parent frame. For example, consider the following frame. The first column of numbers are true positive values (i.e., the fraction of the patients with "Left-sided heart failure" that have the finding) and the second column of numbers are the false positive values (i.e., the fraction of other patients in the population who do not have "Left-sided heart failure" but who do have the finding). (The "•" is a reference to another frame.)

Left-sided heart failure (a priori = .03)		
a. •Left ventricular enlargement	.85	.01
b. •Pulmonary venous congestion	.95	.005
c. •Low cardiac output	.50	.05

If the probability of "Left ventricular enlargement" were 50% at some point in the workup, the effect on the posteriori probability of "Left-sided

heart failure" from processing 0.85 and 0.01 through the Bayes equation
would be reduced (i.e., multiplied by 0.5).

Using Partial Information for Decision Making

"Working up a patient" or making a diagnosis is a problem-solving scenario
in which success depends on the ability of the clinician to form appropriate
hypotheses from partial information as to the nature of the patient's problem at each stage of the process. An expert system must capture the essence
of this algorithm if it is to serve as a source of consultation for the student,
paraprofessional, or physician, or as a standard against which to compare
human decision making.

When a Bayesian frame contains another frame as one of its constituent
complex findings, the effect of the child frame's value on the parent frame
can be calculated using the following empirical relationship[48]:

$$P_{d/f} = \frac{P_d \left(P_{f/d}\right)^a \left(1 - P_{f/d}\right)^b}{P_d \left(P_{f/d}\right)^a \left(1 - P_{f/d}\right)^b + \left(1 - P_d\right)\left(P_{f/nd}\right)^a \left(1 - P_{f/nd}\right)^b}$$

where P_d is the prior probability of the parent frame before considering the
effect of the child frame, $P_{d/f}$ is the posteriori probability of the parent frame
given the partial information about the child frame, $P_{f/d}$ is the sensitivity of
the child frame (i.e., the true positive rate for the child frame in the parent
frame), and $P_{f/nd}$ is the false positive rate (i.e., 1 − specificity) for that
complex finding. The exponential terms a and b (not to be confused with
findings a and b in a frame) are the close_t and close_f values for the child
frame. Note that in the limiting case where a = 1 and b = 0 (or vice versa),
the equation becomes the standard form of Bayes equation for positive or
negative findings.

When a Boolean frame contains complex findings, such as shown here,

---

•Signs and symptoms of anemia
    a. Hx of fatigue
    b. Hx of shortness of breath on exertion
    c. Hx of pallor
    d. PE shows pallor
    e. Heart rate
    f. Hx of palpitations
    g. •Pulse pressure
    h. PE shows ejection murmur
    i. Hx of headache
    j. Recent Hx of anemia
True if (5 of (a, b, (c or d), e > 100, f, g > 50, h, i)) or j

---

then the finding is weighted by its current value. If the logic statement contains a threshold, then the current value of the finding is compared to the threshold to process the logic in the parent frame. So, in "Signs and symptoms of anemia," if the heart rate is 110 this would represent positive information (i.e., 20% of the information necessary to make the frame completely true).

Heuristics That Improve the Model

The Bayesian and Boolean algorithms presented here constitute the basic "inference engine" of the Iliad expert system. On presentation of a set of patient findings, the expert system generates a ranked list of diseases as well as suggestions of additional pertinent information to narrow the list of possibilities. However, after running hundreds of cases through the system, it became apparent that minor adjustments were needed. These heuristics ("rules of thumb") are used to improve the performance of the system in terms of accuracy and user satisfaction.

Risk Flags

One way of preventing diseases from appearing on the differential inappropriately is through the use of risk flags. These are frame-specific flags on findings that essentially say: "Do not process this frame based on this finding alone; wait until more specific information is present." In the following frame, shown with one of its clusters, the findings in item g are flagged with a risk flag (designated by "+"). In other words, if a patient has a "Hx of tuberculosis" (a finding contained in "Risk factors for anemia of chronic disease"), this frame ("Anemia of chronic disease") will not be processed until there is also some evidence of anemia.

Anemia of chronic disease (a priori = .02)		
a. •Anemia	.9999	.10
b. MCHC <32	.49	.09
c. MCV		
<76	.033	.03
76–80	.07	.03
81–85	.23	.04
86–101	.666	.85
≥102	.0005	.05
d. •Serum iron/TIBC (%Fe saturation) <20	.99	.07
e. •Depressed erythropoietic activity	.95	.08
f. Platelet count <140,000	.001	.08
g. +•Risk factors for anemia of chronic disease	.90	.10
or		
+Hx of cancer	.10	.01

h. Serum ferritin <20	.0001	.075
or		
Bone marrow iron absent	.0001	.08
i. Serum TIBC		
<240 µg/dL	.95	.05
240–450	.05	.87
>450	.0001	.08

•Risk factors for anemia of chronic disease
    a. Past Hx of chronic inflammatory disease
    b. Past Hx of chronic infectious disease
    c. Hx of subacute bacterial endocarditis
    d. •Lung abscess
    e. •Pelvic inflammatory disease
    f. Hx of tuberculosis
    g. •Osteomyelitis
    h. Hx of rheumatoid arthritis
    i. Hx of collagen vascular disease
    j. Hx of extensive burns
    k. Hx of AIDS
Value if 1 of (a–k) then true

Display Logic

The Iliad application uses display logic to restrict the appearance of certain diseases on the differential diagnostic list until certain criteria are met. This construct is used primarily to restrict the appearance of common diseases (e.g., common cold) based on nonspecific findings (e.g., fatigue, cough, headache). In the "Viral URI" frame, the patient must have a runny nose or nasal congestion before the frame will appear on the differential.

Viral URI (common cold) (a priori = .01)		
a. Hx of sore throat	.85	.05
or		
Hx of cough	.80	.10
b. Hx of rhinorrhea	.90	.10
or		
Hx of sneezing	.80	.10
or		
Hx of nasal congestion	.90	.10
c. Hx of headache	.90	.15
or		
Hx of myalgia	.80	.05
d. Family Hx of upper respiratory infection, recent	.25	.05
e. Throat culture shows group A, beta-hemolytic		
streptococcal growth	.00001	.05
or		

Streptococcal screen positive	.00001	.05
or		
Throat culture positive for *Neisseria gonorrheae*	.00001	.01

Display logic: b1 or b3

It may be desirable in some cases to have several findings present before displaying the frame on the differential, e.g., display "only if items a and e are present" or "if 2 of (a,b,e,g) are present." If the findings with display flags are themselves clusters, they will have a value associated with them. Bayesian frames have a posteriori probability, Boolean frames have a pseudoprobability (closeness to true or false), and value frames can be true/false or have any numerical value. The display logic of the following frame insists that there be some minimum amount of information about anemia and also about some endocrine disease before the disease appears on the differential.

Anemia of endocrine disease
    a. •Normochromic anemia
    b. •Hypopituitarism
    c. •Hypothyroidism
    d. •Addison's disease
    e. •Testicular failure

True if a and 1 of (b > .50, c > .50, d > .50, e > .50)
Display logic: a ≥ .25 and (b ≥ .3 or c ≥ .3 or d ≥ .3 or e ≥ .3)

Display logic thresholds can be determined by perusing the component frames and empirically trying different likely combinations of data.

It is important to note that, unlike a risk flag or data driver, even when the display logic is not met, the frame is still processed even though it is not displayed. Other frames that use this frame as a complex finding will be calculated and may appear on the differential list, or change their status on the differential, or disappear from the differential as a result. Also, the frames that have not met their display logic criteria will be maintained on an internal differential list so that the system can prompt the user for the necessary data to further evaluate the posteriori value of the frame. The data can be viewed by specifically searching for that frame or by referencing it within another frame that uses it.

Display logic does not usually reference important lab findings specific to that disease, because the tests would probably not have been done unless the disease was strongly suspected in the first place. On the other hand, test batteries (such as Chem20 or CBC) or screening tests (such as CXR or sputum gram stain) might be flagged in some cases if it is likely that a disease would be suddenly suspected as a result of such a test.

Data Drivers

The "data driver" flag and data driver logic demarcate items in a frame that must be true for the frame to be processed (not presently implemented in Iliad). It is similar to the idea of a value frame, except that the frame can be a Bayesian frame, and any combination of findings can be specified. Also, any threshold can be set before which the frame will be processed.

In "Prodrome of measles," all the findings are common and nonspecific. It may then be desirable to require at least two or three of the findings be present before the frame is processed.

Prodrome of measles
  a. Hx of fever >39°C
  b. Hx of cough
  c. Hx of copious nasal discharge
  d. Hx of conjunctivitis

True if a and b and c and d

In "Respiratory distress in a child," appropriate data driver logic might be "a and b" or "a and 1 of (c–h))."

Respiratory distress in a child
  a. Age <10 years
  b. PE shows labored breathing
  c. Respiratory rate >40
  d. PE shows nasal flaring with breathing
  e. PE shows muscle retractions on inspiration
  f. PE shows stridor
  g. PE shows use of accessory muscles of ventilation
  h. PE shows grunting

True if a and b and 1 of (c–h)

In the following frame, it is desirable to have item d be true before allowing the frame to pass information. Having only items a or b or c would produce too many false positives because so many other skin diseases may have papules, plaques, or pustules, and this lesion is one of the least common skin lesions.

Balanitis circinata
  a. PE shows skin lesion with papule
  b. PE shows skin lesion with plaque
  c. PE shows skin lesion with pustule
  d. PE shows skin lesion on penis

        e. PE shows skin lesion with color erythema
        f. PE shows skin lesion with with scale
        g. PE shows skin lesion with with erosion

True if (a or b or c) and d and e and f +/– g

Data driver logic: True if (a or b or c) and d

False positives are even less desirable for frames such as "rash of secondary syphilis" or "Kaposi's sarcoma" or "Alcoholic liver disease," where there is some potential stigma associated with the diagnosis. However, it should be remembered that, if the affected frame is not top level (i.e., a final diagnosis), other controls can be exercised in the parent frame to modulate the effect of a given finding. These would include modifying probabilities, risk flags, or display logic.

The data driver construct would allow the designer of the system to more specifically or selectively determine when a frame should pass information and thereby have a potential effect on the differential diagnostic list. The credibility of the expert system will be strongly affected by the reliability and robustness of the differential list. In this regard, there are several other heuristics that can be programmed into the system. If a frame contains only negative findings, it is usually not desirable to process the frame. In general, this feature will improve the performance of the system.

However, there are some cases in which this rule can cause problems, e.g., if all the items in "Iron deficiency" are negative, no information will be passed. Suppose however that the patient has a type of anemia that is not caused by iron deficiency. "Iron deficiency anemia" will stil be on the differential because it contains the "Anemia" cluster. If no information is passed from the "Iron deficiency" cluster, then "Iron deficiency anemia" will remain on the differential. In the "Iron deficiency" frame below, it can be seen that "Bone marrow iron absent" has been marked with a special flag (δ_2), so that the inference engine can override the default algorithm in this case.

Iron deficiency
a.	Serum ferritin <12 ng/mL	.999	.0001
	or		
	∂_2Bone marrow iron absent	.9999	.0001
b.	Serum TIBC >450 mg/dL	.33	.01
c.	Serum transferrin saturation <20%	.99	.07
d.	RDW >15.3	.90	.30

Iron deficiency anemia (a priori = .075)
a.	•Anemia	.999	.10
b.	•Hypochromic and microcytic RBCs	.85	.07
c.	•Iron deficiency	.9999	.01
	xor		

•At risk for iron deficiency	.95	.25
xor		
•Chronic blood loss	.95	.10
d. •Absolute reticulocyte count		
<50,000	.90	.08
50,000–200,000	.10	.84
≥200,000	.001	.08
e. •Thalassemia minor	.0008	.008

This type of flag should probably be transparent to the user, while risk flags, data drivers, and display logic should be accessible by the interested user to explain a frame's behavior in various circumstances.

False positives can cause inappropriate diseases to appear on the differential and seriously compromise the credibility of the system. Double negatives are a common potential source of false positives. For example, in the following frame, the absence of "Chronic myelomonocytic leukemia" by itself should not put "RAEB" on the differential with a probability of .33 (as item c represents 1/3 of the information required to make the frame completely true). Such double negatives must be formally excluded by the inference engine.

RAEB (refractory anemia with excess blasts)
  a. •Myelodysplastic syndrome
  b. •Marrow and blood differential of RAEB
  c. •Chronic myelomonocytic leukemia

True if a and b and not c

4
The Data Dictionary: Limiting the Domain of the Model

The data dictionary of an expert system is the component that describes all the terms known to the system. In a diagnostic expert system, the data dictionary is the set of diseases and disease manifestations (i.e., symptoms, signs, laboratory results, radiological results, and special procedures) across all the diseases represented in the knowledge base.

Organization of the Dictionary

The data dictionary for a medical expert system can potentially be constructed in a number of different ways. What constraints or criteria should be used to help guide the design of the dictionary and what priorities should be assigned to each when trade-offs need to be made? Information should be organized in a way that makes good medical sense, e.g., separating symptoms, signs, lab results, and imaging. The dictionary can be organized to optimize inferencing, searching, data entry, ease of management, etc. Good organization can simultaneously facilitate management, data entry, and searching. Whatever the organization, it is important to avoid representing the same term multiple times by phrasing it in different ways. On the other hand, the same phrase, in a different context, may represent a different term or concept.

Context Versus Concept

The dictionary may be organized so that the context is separate from concepts. For example, consider the following findings:

Family history of pneumonia
Past history of pneumonia
Present history of pneumonia

There is one clinical concept and three contexts.

The concept "penicillin" could be used in the context of a currently administered drug, a drug level, a drug allergy, or a microbial sensitivity. Each of these contexts corresponds to a separate hierarchy in the data dictionary.

Hierarchical Relationships

Medical terminology is naturally hierarchical. Some example hierarchical segments are shown here:

Hx of cough
   that is productive
     of purulent sputum

Hx of abdominal pain
   [with location]
     in the RUQ
   [with time pattern]
     with onset 2 months ago
     recurring
     with episodes that last for 2 hours
     that is colicky
   [with severity]
     mild
     moderate
     moderate to severe
     severe
   [aggravated by]
     fatty foods
   [relieved by]
     fasting
     analgesics

PE shows swelling
   of the knee
     on the right side
     that is extensive
     that has been present for 2 weeks
     associated with an injury to the knee

PE of skin shows rash/lesion
   [primary characteristic (lesion type)] that is a
     bullae
     burrow
     comedone
     cyst

      infarct
      macule
      nodule
      patch
      papule
         that is dome-shaped
         that is flat-topped
         that is umbilicated
         that is verrucous

Microbiology shows
  sputum culture
    positive for *Staphylococcus aureus*
      that is sensitive to penicillin

CXR shows
  parenchymal lesion
    opacity(ies)
      [location/distribution]
        anterior
        bilateral
          symmetrical
        posterior
        left
        right
        —
        localized
        diffuse/extensive
        adjacent to the pleural surface
        —
        apical
        peripheral
        perihilar
        —
        lobar
        whole lung
        lower lung zone
        middle lung zone
        upper lung zone
        segmental
        changed in location since last film
      [size]
        diameter—(cm)
        large and small
        uniform
      multiple

[descriptor]
   calcified
   cavitated
      containing a mobile rounded opacity
      thick-walled
   confluent
   migratory
   paired line ("tram-tracks")
   poorly marginated
   reticular (small, irregular)
   rounded
   septal (Kerley) line(s)
   spiculated
   triangular
   tubular ("gloved fingers")
   well-circumscribed
   with retraction
   with scarring
mass(es)

Granularity of the Dictionary

Granularity of the dictionary should be appropriate to the sophistication of the system. Granularity refers to the size of the "chunks" or items in the dictionary. For example, chest pain could be defined as two separate items or concepts (high granularity) or as a single concept (lower granularity). The combined term is sometimes referred to as a "molecule," and the individual items can be referred to as "atoms." The higher the granularity, the more flexible the dictionary is in the sense that the items can be combined in any conceivable way as complex terms. However, increased granularity usually equates to higher complexity in terms of designing and using the expert system. The level of granularity should be in line with the intended use of the system.

A decision must be made at the outset whether to only allow as many hierarchical levels as necessary to support the frames currently in the knowledge base (and then to add to the hierarchy as necessary) or whether to build an elaborate comprehensive structure that would allow for any conceivable future addition. In either case, there will obviously be an uneven depth distribution because some findings have more qualifiers/descriptors than others.

For certain situations, it may be desirable to have additional hierarchies that serve special purposes. For example, a drug hierarchy may be associated with the system that includes drugs not referenced by frames currently in the system. This would allow the user to enter a drug from this ancillary hierarchy, which could be determined to be equivalent to a drug actually used in a frame by a mapping table. Alternatively, a dialogue could inform the user that it is not in the system and suggest alternatives, or the user could be allowed to get information about that drug even though it would not drive the expert system.

Modifying the Dictionary

In general, we recommend that terms only be included in the dictionary that are used in frames in the knowledge base. Terms are then added as needed. In this case, the dictionary program itself must allow for new terms to be put into the appropriate place in the hierarchy. Obviously, if adding new terms changed preexisting dictionary codes, then cases run with previous versions of the dictionary would not run correctly. Therefore, it is necessary to have some absolute number associated with each finding (i.e., a unique identifier in a "master object index"[49] that does not vary as the system changes [they may be referred to, e.g., as CIDs (concept identifiers) or EIDS (expression identifiers)]. These identifiers may be associated with hierarchical codes that can be used by the inference engine at runtime. Multiple codes representing multiple subhierarchies of the dictionary may be used as needed (independent of the unique identifier) to facilitate data entry, display, and inferencing.

Knowledge Contained in the Dictionary

An enormous amount of inherent information can be stored within the structure of the dictionary hierarchy. The numbers of hierarchies and naming conventions are important. For example, level 1 categories might be "Past Hx," "Family Hx," "Occupational and Environmental Hx," "Social Hx," "Present Hx," "Physical exam," "Laboratory," "Imaging," "Diagnostic procedures," or "Diagnostic frames." For a simpler system, all the history levels could be subsumed under a "Symptoms of" level.

Iliad uses a six-part hierarchical code. For example:

1.0.0.0.0.0:	Present history
1.5.0.0.0.0	General symptoms:
1.5.2.0.0.0	fever
1.5.2.15.0.0	[quality]
1.5.2.15.2.0	low grade (101F or 38C or lower)
1.5.2.15.4.0	high grade (102F or 38.5C or higher)
1.5.2.20.0.0	[time pattern]
1.5.2.20.2.0	for—weeks

| 1.5.2.20.4.0 | increasing |
| 1.5.2.20.4.5 | rapidly |

Consistency of structure and terminology within the dictionary is important in terms of maintenance and the user interface. For example, wherever possible under major symptoms, it is advisable to use a standard set of subcategories wherever it is appropriate, e.g., "Location," "Time pattern," "Severity," "Aggravating factors," and "Relieving factors."

Each term in the dictionary should have an associated list of keywords that facilitate retrieval by the user. Some expert systems include a facility to delete stop words and to ignore or delete certain suffixes. It is advisable to include common abbreviations and possibly misspellings. It is assumed that the users will be informed at some point in their training whether searching is case sensitive, whether the order of the words is important, and whether parts of words are acceptable search terms. Although this is a software interface rather than a dictionary issue per se, such criteria should always be kept in mind when designing the dictionary and assigning keywords to the findings. Increased richness of the keywords facilitates data retrieval and diminishes frustration on the part of the user. Performance is rarely an issue with current hardware. One caveat should be mentioned, however. Keywords should be assigned at the appropriate levels of the dictionary, e.g., "muscle" should not be assigned as a keyword for "Musculoskeletal symptoms" because it would retrieve everything in that hierarchy including all the joint symptoms that have nothing to do with muscles in this context.

Other kinds of knowledge can be included directly in the dictionary.[36] For example, the frequency at which a given finding appears in the population of interest could be stored in the dictionary and retrieved at runtime. There may also be various flags on each finding that essentially restrict the use of a finding to particular situations, e.g., numerical item, yes/no item (see also data relations, word relations, risk flags, display flags, data drivers).

Inferencing from the Hierarchy

Inferencing within the dictionary makes use of the inherent relationships among the terms in the dictionary to facilitate data entry and processing. Consider the following hierarchy segment:

CXR shows
  parenchymal lesion
    opacity(ies)
      [descriptor]
        calcified
        cavitated

    and containing a mobile rounded opacity
    thick-walled
    thin-walled
  confluent
[location/distribution]

If the user enters a "yes" for "thick-walled," the system should assume a "yes" for all the parents of that term, i.e., cavitated, opacity, and parenchymal lesion. All frames that use those parent terms, in addition to the more specific one ("thick-walled"), would then be processed by the inference engine. On the other hand, if the user entered a "no" for "thick-walled," the system should not necessarily assume a "no" for any of its parents. In other words, "yes"s, but not "no"s, propagate up the hierarchy.

It is also true that "no"s propagate down the hierarchy. If the user enters a "no" for "parenchymal lesion" on CXR, all its child findings can immediately be inferred to be "no" and all frames containing those findings should be processed accordingly. In other words, "no"s, but not "yes"s, propagate down the hierarchy.

It is theoretically possible to propagate "no"s up the hierarchy to some extent. For example, suppose it was known that in a given population, 20% of the parenchymal cavitated opacities were thick-walled, 10% thin-walled, and 70% in between. Suppose the user entered a "no" for thick-walled. As thick-walled comprise 1/5 of all the cavitated opacities, there is then a 20% chance of a "no" for cavitated opacity.

Another concept ("the **inferred no**") is worth mentioning at this juncture, because although it is primarily a user interface or software design issue it can have a large effect on the efficacy of an expert system. Consider the following hierarchy segment:

PE of skin shows rash/lesion
  [primary characteristic (lesion type)] that is/is a
    bullae
    burrow
    comedone
    cyst
    infarct
    macule
    nodule
    patch
    papule
      that is dome-shaped
      that is flat-topped
      that is umbilicated
      that is verrucous
    petechiae
    plaque

    pustule
    sinus tract drainage
    spider telangiectasia
    striae
    tumor
    vesicle (blister)
    wheal
[color]
    brown/tan
    erythema
    flesh-colored
    golden-yellow (honey-colored)
    hypopigmentation
      white (depigmented)
    hyperpigmentation
    red/brown
    salmon
    trichrome (three-colored)
    violaceous
[border]
    active
    diffuse
    irregular
    raised "pearly"
    sharp/distinct

Suppose the user describes a lesion as an erythematous rash with macules and papules and distinct borders. Can we assume "no"s to all the other findings in the "primary characteristic," "color," and "border" categories, because the physician probably would have entered those findings if they were there? The answer may depend on which hierarchy and who the user is. The decision is easy to make in some cases. For example, "Renal biopsy shows. . . ." This is likely a relatively small set of findings, and we can feel quite safe in assuming the user would have perused all the possible entries and marked all the ones that were positive. However, this will depend, to some extent, on the mode the user uses to enter the data. If the user is using keywords, some keywords might pull up only part of the findings in the set. Ideally, it would be preferable only to use the "inferred no" if the user enters data in a mode in which we can be assured that they have seen all the entries. This would also decrease the uncertainty associated with having users who are more or less familiar with the software and its dictionary. The software could provide the user the option of turning the "inferred no" option on or off with a "Preferences" dialog. In any event, the software must provide the user a way of viewing the inferred "no"s and subsequently changing their mind about those findings.

To incorporate inferred "no"s in an expert system, appropriate hierarchies need to be flagged in the dictionary *at the appropriate level*. This is a task that must be done carefully. If the hierarchy is too large, e.g., "CXR shows" or even "CXR shows a parenchymal abnormality," it is likely that the user will enter some data without wading through all the questions. So, in this example, "inferred no" flags should be placed in the dictionary at a lower level in the hierarchy.

Word Relations

Other relationships in addition to hierarchical parent–child relationships can be stored in the dictionary or in separate files. In Iliad, a special WordRelations file (see Appendix 6) facilitates searching for related terms [e.g., (1) entering the keyword "white blood cell" will retrieve all the related findings: "WBC," "leukocytes," "leukopenia," "leukocytosis," etc.; (2) entering "color" retrieves red, green, yellow, etc.]. This construct increases the number of findings returned when the user enters a keyword or keywords. However, if it used inappropriately, the user will be overwhelmed with numerous inappropriate findings (e.g., "joint" is related to "bone" in some cases, but not often enough to justify a word relation).

Data Relations

Iliad makes use of a special construct called DataRelations (see Appendix 5), which presently allows three types of relationships (others would be desirable):

1. **Not applicable:** If the first finding in a group is positive, then all the other findings in the same group will be not applicable (N/A) and omitted from the display, e.g.,
   If "Hx of splenectomy" is true, then "Abdominal ultrasound shows enlarged spleen," "CT shows enlarged spleen," "MRI shows enlarged spleen," and "CXR shows enlarged spleen" are inferred to N/A.
   If Sex is male, then all findings associated with menstrual period are N/A.
2. **Mutually exclusive:** Only one finding can be true in the same group, e.g.,
   If "sex, male" then "sex, female" is inferred to false.
   If "PE shows eye discharge" is true then "PE shows dry eyes" is inferred to false.
   If "PE shows hypoactive bowel sounds" is true then "PE of borborygmus" and "PE of absent of bowel sounds" are inferred to false.
   If blood group is A, then blood group is not B, AB, or O.
3. **Same value:** All the findings in a given group have the same value, e.g.,

If "PE shows a distended abdomen" is true then "Hx of abdominal distension" is inferred to true.

If "Chem20" gives a glucose value, the "Chem7" glucose may be assigned the same value.

If "Sigmoidoscopy shows polyp', then "Colonoscopy shows polyp."

Note that the last example is not really accurate. Because sigmoidoscopy only looks at part of the colon, it is theoretically possible to see a polyp by colonoscopy but not by sigmoidoscopy. In practice, this probably does not happen because if there were polyps in the sigmoid colon, then there would probably also be polyps in other parts of the colon. Nevertheless, it would be preferable to have "Same value" relationships that only go in one direction, i.e., from the specific to the general and not the other way around. It would also be desirable to have a relationship similar to a "mutually exclusive" relationship where some combination of items in a group can simultaneously be true, e.g., (1) several biopsy findings may be seen simultaneously, while others may never be seen together; or (2) certain gram-negative rods or cocci may coexist, while others are never seen together.

5
The Knowledge Engineering Process

How to Structure/Model the Knowledge

In a diagnostic medical expert system it is wise to make certain decisions before jumping into the details of designing individual frames. For example:

•For what purpose is the expert system being designed?
•Who will the primary users be?
•What are the limits of the medical domain to be modeled? This will affect the size and organization of the dictionary and data entry by the user.
•What is the patient population? The patient population will determine the a prioris and specificities to be used in the frames.
•How difficult it is to get the probability estimates?
•What experts are available?
•Approximately how much time and effort will be required to complete the initial construction of the knowledge base?
•Approximately how much time and effort will be required to test and evaluate the system, and what resources are available for the effort?

The Overall Process

The basic steps in constructing the knowledge base are as follow:

•Construct a list or hierarchy of the top-level diagnoses or decisions to be included in the knowledge base
•As each frame is constructed, decide which findings are pertinent to that disease
•Decide whether to model each frame as a Bayesian or Boolean frame
•Decide which elements of the frame are complex findings and define the relevant clusters (use preexisting clusters when possible)

- Define the organization of elements within the frame, especially which findings should be "or"ed together in Bayesian frames
- Obtain or estimate prevalence, sensitivities, and specificities for Bayesian frames
- Determine logic for Boolean frames
- Test the frames in isolation using a Bayesian or Boolean calculator if one is available
- Translate the findings in each new frame into the elements of a structured dictionary
- Generate precompiled frames with structured dictionary elements
- Compile the frames together into a form that optimizes execution by the inference engine
- Test the frames within the context of the whole expert system
- Make modifications to the original frames and repeat the cycle whenever problems are found during testing

The system must ultimately be tested in the working environment where it was designed to be used. Some of the questions that may arise when this is done include the following:

- Does the keyword entry accommodate the needs of the users? The user may have trouble finding the keyword needed to enter a concept.
- Is there more than one way to express a given concept in the structured vocabulary? This kind of error may be discovered when a user enters a concept and finds that it did not drive a frame they expected it might.
- Does it take more time to enter the data than is acceptable to the prospective user?
- Does the differential diagnosis make suggestions that are useful and appropriate at each stage of the workup? Does the user develop confidence in the suggestions made as they get more experience with the system?
- Does the "best information" algorithm improve the efficiency of the workup?
- How much training is required before a user can use the system to maximum advantage?

Knowledge Sources: Advantages and Limitations of Each

Literature

The medical literature can be useful in determining important criteria to include in a diagnostic frame. Published criteria for a number of common disorders have been put forward by various medical organizations. Prevalence data are frequently available in the literature, sensitivities (true positive rates) are sometimes available, and specificities (false positive rates) are rarely available. However, even when desired probabilities are found, there are often questions about the size of the study and whether the control and patient populations were comparable to the population for which an expert system is being designed. Clinical population studied are usually limited because of constraints on available resources, time, personnel, and money. Also, many studies do not collect the kinds of quantitative data that would be useful for an expert system. Combining multiple studies introduces additional sources of ambiguity because of differences in selection criteria, parameters measured, methodologies, etc.

Patient Data Repositories

Data obtained from a patient database are valuable when available. However, even when these data are available, they are usually incomplete. Few institutions have routinely collected history and physical exam data in electronic form. When they do, it is usually unstructured and incomplete information. Manual chart review may be an option, but the data are inevitably incomplete or phrased in a wide variety of ways. Many approximations and interpretations are necessary to extract the data, so the uncertainties associated with the final result are very significant. If the domain of the expert system is a relatively restricted subset, adequate data may be available in a particular clinic for common disorders. Statistically significant data for rare disorders will most likely not be available.

Certain laboratory and imaging studies and various procedures may be done routinely as part of standard operating procedures in the hospital in general or in particular clinics. For example, patients admitted to a cardiology service will likely have an ECG and possibly ECHO studies done; patients in hematology will have CBC data; pulmonary patients will have spirometry and blood gas measurements. Any data that are available can be used in combination with estimates of the missing data to get initial approximations, which can then be refined through an iterative process with the help of experts and by testing and evaluating the sytems performance as described elsewhere in this book.

When seeking data to estimate the sensitivity of a finding from a patient database for use in an expert system, it should be kept in mind that the patients who have the data are usually preselected. Specificities are not usually available because in general not all patients were tested for the finding. Approximations can be made based on the assumption that untested patients would be "normal" or that their data values would be normally distributed. When such approximations are made, a vigorous effort should be made to use the same approximations and assumptions consistently in the knowledge base wherever applicable. If an estimate is later adjusted, it should be changed in all frames that make use of it.

The reliability of the data can be increased by using thresholds well outside the normal range to separate the disease from the nondisease

population. For example, the normal ranges of serum AST and ALT are
10–34 U/L and 6–59 U/L, respectively (in our local lab); however, hepatitis
patients may have values over 1000. The disease threshold can be phrased
as 2× the ULN (upper limit of normal) or some other appropriate multiple.
Multiple bins with different thresholds are another option:

d. •Absolute reticulocyte count		
<50,000	.90	.08
50,000–200,000	.10	.84
≥200,000	.001	.08

Expert Opinion

Expert estimates are the most accessible, but probably the least reliable,
source of probabilities. Because the reliability of such estimates is dependent on the experience of the expert, they are generally more accurate for
the more common diseases and findings. It is essential that the experts
understand the meaning of the probabilities they are attempting to estimate. For example, the meaning of sensitivity (i.e., the true positive rate of
a finding) can be explained to the medical expert by asking: "How many of
the last 100 patients you saw in whom you diagnosed this disease had this
symptom at the time you first made the diagnosis?" Frequently, heuristics
will have to be resorted to for rare conditions, e.g., by making comparisons
to other diseases and findings where the numbers are more certain. For
example, the expert might be asked to compare the sensitivity of a finding
that he or she is having trouble estimating with the previously determined
sensitivity of another finding in that disease. Combining the results of
multiple experts in a consensus fashion will improve the reliability of the
data.

   Obviously, the term "expert" could be defined in various ways. A clinician who specializes in rheumatology, for example, would be considered
an expert in joint disease but not in other specialties. However, a
rheumatologist who has been in the field for 30 years may have seen
hundreds of patients with a particular disease, while a new staff member
may have seen only a few. Even the most experienced specialist will not
have seen patients with all diseases in a given specialty as some diseases are
extremely rare.

Which Findings to Include in a Frame

Diagnostic frames are a collection of findings pertinent to making a diagnosis of a particular disease. The frame includes the relationships of the
findings to the disease and the findings to each other.

How does one decide whether or not to include a given finding in a frame? At least three reasons for including findings in a frame can be stated:

1. The finding occurs frequently in patients with the disease; it is necessary or important for diagnostic purposes, i.e., the expert uses it.

2. The finding occurs infrequently in patients with the disease but has a high specificity (i.e., it rarely occurs in people who do not have the disease). For example, a finding of anterior lenticonus on ophthalmic exam is rarely encountered in patients with Alport syndrome, but if it is present, it is almost pathognomonic for the disease (because it is essentially nonexistent in other diseases).

3. The finding never occurs in this disease and its presence rules out the disease.

One must find a happy medium between having only really pertinent findings and having so many findings that the frame becomes overwhelmingly complicated and difficult to follow. A frame that is too sparse will have limited educational value. It will also perform poorly in a simulation mode because the diagnosis will be made on the basis of only a few findings. In addition, because some kinds of data can be obtained in more than one way [e.g., (i) "History of muscular weakness" and "PE shows muscular weakness"; (ii) "polyuria" and "increased urine volume"], the related findings would ordinarily all be positive or negative. However, this may not be the case if one method is more sensitive than another or if observations are significantly separated in time. Each disease should ideally have associated with it all clinical data that are relevant and ordinarily used to diagnose that disease in practice.

One way of avoiding the complexity associated with a long list of findings is to group some of the findings into clusters (i.e., subframes representing intermediate decisions). The use of clusters is also one strategy to minimize overconfidence from an accumulated effect of dependent findings (the other strategy is with the use of the "or" construct) (see Chapter 3).

Probabilistic and Deterministic Logic

Bayesian frames take into account the prevalence of a disease and also the uncertainty of relations between a disease and its findings. They also give more realistic estimates of the degree of certainty of an expert when only partial imformation is available early in the case. However, the required statistics may be difficult or impossible to acquire or the findings may be closely related (and therefore not independent). "Top-level" diseases (i.e., final diagnoses) are usually modeled as Bayesian frames unless Boolean criteria have been well established and are currently accepted in practice (e.g., diagnosis of AIDS, lupus erythematosus, rheumatoid arthritis, multiple myeloma, or Rett's syndrome). Such Boolean criteria emanate from published guidelines, e.g., from the American Rheumatology Association, the American Heart Association, Agency for Health Care Policy and Research (AHCPR), or DSM-IV.[38]

There are some exceptional cases in which top-level deterministic frames may be desirable for heuristic reasons, e.g., COPD (chronic obstructive pulmonary disease) and heart failure, but in all these cases, probabilistic frames are used as data items in the top level Boolean frame as illustrated here:

Chronic obstructive pulmonary disease
    a. Chronic bronchitis
    b. Emphysema
True if a or b
Heart failure
    a. Left-sided heart failure
    b. Right-sided heart failure
True if a or b

These frames work satisfactorily because of the special form of the simplistic logic and the fact that the constituent clusters are Bayesian. Each of these clusters passes partial information (see Chapter 3) up to the parent frame, which then uses whichever finding has the highest value, be it positive or negative.

Reasons to Cluster

There are some general reasons to group findings into clusters:

1. Grouping reduces the size of the frame and thereby makes it easier to comprehend (although excessive nesting can make it more difficult to comprehend).

2. The constituent findings are related because they result from some common underlying pathophysiological process [e.g., "Lung consolidation" (see below) or "Wernicke's aphasia" (see below)]. This construct makes the frame easier to understand and increases its educational value.

3. Numerous studies have shown that experts make use of bigger "chunks" of information than novices.[47,50] The use of clusters allows the expert system to more closely mimic the behavior of experts.

4. A common collection of findings being used by a number of frames (e.g., signs of systemic infection) may be combined into a cluster. This decreases the size of the expert system and simultaneously makes its performance more efficient. It also ensures consistency between related or competing frames in their use of findings or statistics.

5. Boolean clusters are a means to isolate dependent findings from a Bayesian frame (sequential Bayes requires that findings be largely indepedent to avoid overconfidence).

6. If all the findings in a cluster are negative, a much more powerful "no" can be passed up the diagnostic hierarchy than if only some of the findings in the cluster are negative.

Lung consolidation
   a. PE shows abnormal chest percussion with dullness
   b. PE shows abnormal pulmonary auscultation with bronchial breath sounds
   c. PE shows abnormal pulmonary auscultation with egophony
      (E-to-A changes)
   d. PE shows abnormal chest palpation with increased vocal
      fremitus
   e. PE shows abnormal pulmonary auscultation with rales
   f. PE shows abnormal pulmonary auscultation with
      pectoriloquy
True if (a or b) and 2 of (c,d,e,f)

Wernicke's aphasia
   a. PE shows impaired comprehension of written/spoken word
   b. PE shows speech that is fluent with paraphrasia and neologisms
   c. PE shows inability to repeat sounds and words
   d. PE shows naming of objects is impaired
   e. PE shows alexia
   f. PE shows agraphia
True if a and b and c and (d or e or f)

Findings may be dependent for several reasons:

1. One item may be a more specific case of another, e.g., cough and productive cough
2. Multiple findings that relate to the same pathophysiological process may change concurrently; e.g., serum urea, creatinine, and phosphate are all increased in renal failure as a result of compromised tubular function
3. The same pathology may be shown by different tests

Nonindependence is usually present for (a) situations in which two findings are in the same hierarchy of the data dictionary, and (b) where one finding is contingent on another finding (e.g., female gender and pregnancy). In other cases the findings are nearly synonymous, but are obtained by different methods or are separated in time.

In many cases, the nonindependence is less obvious. These are usually cases in which the relationship is a causal one. Generally, the two findings are the result of the same pathophysiological process (e.g., elevated WBCs and fever resulting from an inflammatory process). This generally decreases diagnostic accuracy, unless it can somehow be compensated.

Some kinds of nonindependence can be handled within a parent Bayesian frame using the "or" construct (see Chapter 3), e.g.:

Iron deficiency anemia (a priori = .075)		
a. Anemia	.999	.10
b. Hypochromic and microcytic RBCs	.85	.07
c. Iron deficiency	.9999	.01
xor		
At risk for iron deficiency	.95	.25
xor		
Chronic blood loss	.95	.10
d. Absolute reticulocyte count		
<50,000	.90	.08
50,000–200,000	.10	.84
≥200,000	.001	.08

Recall that the "xor" allows negative findings to override positive findings, while the "or" (sometimes designated "nor") always uses positive information over negative information. The "or" (or "xor") method is appropriate when the list of related findings is fairly short and when good estimates for sensitivities and specificities are available. This may be the best method when nonindependent findings have sensitivities and specificities that are very different from one another. A variation of this construct with a series of bins (e.g., absolute reticulocyte count in "Iron deficiency anemia" or WBC in "hairy cell leukemia") can be used to model a graded difference in statistical weights. Although the performance of frames using this construct is frequently acceptable, there are probably cases where the treatment of partial independence with a more sophisticated model would be beneficial.

Hairy cell leukemia (a priori = .000003)		
a. Sex, male	.83	.55
b. Age >40 years	.90	.70
c. Enlarged spleen	.81	.04
d. Enlarged liver by PE	.24	.07
e. Clinical evidence of hemostatic defect	.24	.02
or		
Thrombocytopenia	.95	.08
f. Lymphadenopathy	.19	.05
g. Hx of fatigue	.51	.20
or		
Anemia	.75	.17
h. Hx of sweating at night	.20	.10
i. WBC		
<5000	.64	.03
5000–10,000	.18	.90
>10,000	.18	.07

j. Differential shows hairy cells	.91	.01
or		
Differential shows hairy cells confirmed by		
TRAP (tartrate-resistant acid phosphatase) stain	.95	.00001
or		
Bone marrow biopsy shows hairy cells	.999	.0000001

On the other hand, a special advantage of using a cluster to represent a series of findings that measure the same thing is that the absence of any or all the items can be used as a strong negative in the parent frame, e.g., "Cough pattern of bronchiectasis" in "Bronchiectasis":

Bronchiectasis (a priori = .0009)		
a. Age <40 years	.85	.41
b. •Predisposing factors for bronchiectasis	.50	.01
or		
Hx of multiple, recurrent upper respiratory infections	.20	.03
or		
Hx of recurrent pneumonia	.40	.02
or		
Hx of slowly resolving pneumonia	.40	.02
or		
Hx of recurrent sinusitis	.40	.025
c. •Cough pattern of bronchiectasis	.999	.01
xor		
Hx of foul sputum production	.10	.005
xor		
Hx of cough with blood-streaked sputum	.80	.007
xor		
Hx of cough with gross hemoptysis	.20	.001
xor		
Hx of cough worse lying on one side	.20	.02
e. PE shows nail abnormalities with clubbing	.07	.05
f. Pulmonary auscultation with rales in lower lung fields	.40	.15
g. •CXR signs of bronchiectasis	.15	.01
or		
Bronchogram shows bronchiectasis	.99	.001
or		
CT scan of chest shows bronchiectasis	.55	.001
h. Sputum gram stain shows bacteria	.975	.15

Types of Clusters

As noted in the previous section, one motivation for constructing clusters is to simplify the presentation of the parent frame and to group findings into convenient pieces that are at the same time educational and easier to understand. For example, signs (i.e., physical exam findings) may be grouped into a cluster:

Exam findings of pneumothorax
    a. PE shows unilateral chest hyperresonance to percussion
    b. PE shows unilateral decreased breath sounds
    c. PE shows unilateral chest hyperinflation
    d. PE shows decreased chest motion unilaterally
    e. PE shows unilateral dullness
True if a and (b or c or d) and not e

This reduces overconfidence in the parent frame (i.e., the frame using the cluster as a complex finding) and can make the parent frame easier to understand when there are many related signs.

Signs and symptoms may be grouped in a common cluster, especially if the logic is "True if any" or if all the elements have approximately the same weight:

Signs and symptoms of neuroglycopenia
    a. Hx of episodic confusion
    b. Hx of amnesia
    c. PE shows confusion
    d. PE shows stupor
    e. PE shows coma
    f. PE shows seizure
True if any

When and how to group signs and symptoms into clusters is up to the discretion of the expert and the knowledge engineer. The organization should make sense clinically. Usually, there are multiple ways of organizing the findings. Clustering of signs and symptoms in Iliad has not been done entirely consistently.

A cluster may be a description or interpretation of a method or procedure:

Positive PPD skin test
    a. PPD = = = (mm diameter)
    b. Second strength PPD (250 TU) = = = (mm diameter)
    c. History of BCG vaccination
True if ((a ≥ 10 or ((a > 6 and a < 10) and b > 10)) and not c

ECG consistent with cor pulmonale
    a. ECG shows right ventricular hypertrophy

   b. ECG shows right bundle branch block
   c. ECG shows right axis deviation
   d. ECG shows right atrial enlargement
   e. ECG shows clockwise rotation of the precordial axis
True if a or b or 2 of (c,d,e)

CXR signs of bronchiectasis
   a. CXR shows tubular shadows or paired line shadows
   b. CXR shows rounded and irregularly nodular densities
   c. CXR shows "gloved-finger shadows" (mucoid impacted bronchi)
   d. CXR shows cystic spaces
   e. CXR shows alveolar infiltrate
True if 2 of (a–e)

A cluster may be composed of different methods for obtaining the same result:

Culture positive for Mycobacterium tuberculosis
   a. Sputum culture positive for *Mycobacterium tuberculosis*
   b. Gastric aspirate culture positive for *Mycobacterium tuberculosis*
   c. Urine culture positive for *Mycobacterium tuberculosis*
   d. Lung biopsy specimen positive for *Mycobacterium tuberculosis*
   e. Bronchial lavage culture positive for *Mycobacterium tuberculosis*
True if a or b or c or d or e

A cluster is a convenient way of grouping a list of risk factors:

At risk for loss of diabetic control
   a. •Acute severe illness
   b. Hx of discontinuance of insulin
   c. Hx of discontinuance of sulfonylurea therapy
True if any

At risk for primary lung cancer
   a. Hx of cigarette smoking for >20 pack-yrs
   b. Hx of chronic bronchitis
   c. Hx of emphysema
   d. •Asbestos exposure
   e. Hx of exposure to uranium dust
   f. Hx of exposure to ionizing radiation
   g. •Nickel exposure
   h. Hx of exposure to chlormethyl methyl ether
   i. •Chromium exposure
   j. •Arsenic exposure
   k. Family Hx of lung cancer
   l. CXR shows old scar
True if any

In the foregoing example, any one of the findings is sufficient to satisfy the logic, even though the findings may be of widely different weights. However, if the weights are available and pertinent, a Bayesian risk cluster can be constructed.

High risk factors for hepatitis B (a priori = .001)
a. Homosexual male	.10	.005
or		
Hx of being an intravenous drug user	.20	.003
or		
•Hemophilia or other coagulation disorder	.04	.00004
or		
Hx of current dialysis treatment	.04	.00004
or		
Hx of recent transfusion of blood or components (>6 units)	.05	.005
or		
Hx of occupational exposure to blood or blood products	.05	.0025
or		
Hx of heterosexual contact with hepatitis B risk group	.70	.0005
or		
Hx of child with mother at risk for hepatitis B	.085	.00002

A cluster may contain a list of possible etiologies of some disease process. Examples of this type include "causes of" frames, "predisposing factor" frames, "exposure" frames, and "occupational history" frames:

Causes of ectopic SIADH (syndrome of inappropriate ADH secretion)
   a. Hx of pulmonary tuberculosis
   b. Hx of current lung abscess
   c. Hx of lymphosarcomas
   d. Hx of pancreatic tumor
   e. Hx of oat cell carcinoma of the lung
   f. Hx of thymoma
True if any

Predisposing factors for bronchiectasis
   a. Hx of pneumonia in infancy or childhood
   b. Hx of foreign body aspiration
   c. Past Hx of congenital agammaglobulinemia (Bruton's type)
   d. Past Hx of acquired IgG deficiency
   e. Immunoglobulin electrophoresis shows selective deficiency of an IgG subclass
   f. Hx of immotile cilia syndrome
True if any

Exposure to high concentrations of silica
   a. Occupational Hx of tunneling for ≥2 yr

  b. Occupational Hx of quarrying for ≥2 yr
  c. Occupational Hx of sand blasting for ≥2 yr
  d. Occupational Hx of lens grinding for ≥2 yr
  e. Occupational Hx of work in manufacturing abrasive soap for ≥2 yr
True if any

Clusters may be used to describe the consequences of a primary disease process, e.g., "Diabetic nephropathy" and "Complications of vomiting":

       <u>Complications of recurrent vomiting</u>
         c. PE shows parotid enlargement
         d. PE shows dental enamel erosion
         e. Serum potassium (mEq/L)
         f. •Hypochloremic metabolic alkalosis
       True if a or b or (c < 3.5 and d)

Clusters are a convenient way to group a list of microorganisms or drugs with something in common:

<u>Culture positive for organisms important in hospital-acquired pneumonias</u>
Culture positive for . . .
  a. *E. coli*
  b. *Pseudomonas*
  c. *Hemophilus*
  d. *Klebsiella*
  e. *Anaerobic bacteria*
  f. *Staphylococcus aureus*
  g. *Enterobacter*
  h. *Providencia*
  i. *Acinetobacter*
  j. *Serratia*
True if any

<u>Drugs causing nephrotoxicity</u>
  a. Hx of recent aminoglycoside antibiotics administration for >7 days
  b. Hx of recent aminoglycoside antibiotics administration at doses inappropriately high for degree of renal dysfunction
  c. Hx of current use of NSAIDs
  d. Hx of current use of amphotericin
  e. Hx of current use of cyclosporine
  f. Hx of recent intravascular radiocontrast agent
True if 1 of a–f

Frames That Return a Value

Besides Bayesian and Boolean frames, there are also value (i.e., calculation) frames that return either a logical or numeric answer:

High serum, low urine osmolality
   a. Serum osmolality
   b. Calculated serum osmolality
   c. Urine osmolality
   d. Urine specific gravity .
Value if (a > 300 or b > 300) and (c < 200 or d < 1.005) then true

---

This frame returns a value of true or false. Note that all findings are required to be present. In other words, value frames do not pass partial information. If one of the findings in a value frame is a probabilistic cluster, it must have a threshold to determine whether a constituent finding is yes or no; a default threshold of .95 may be used.

An example of a value frame that returns a numerical value follows:

Calculated serum osmolality
   a. Serum Na^+
   b. Serum glucose
   c. BUN
Value if all then $1.86*a + b/18 + c/2.8$

Value frames can include complicated relationships:

Serum cholesterol (predicted)
   a. Sex (male)
   b. Age
Value if a then $(66.9 + 5.49*b - .0602*b^2 + .00017*b^3)$ or if not a then $(179 - 2.6*b + .11*b^2 - .00086*b^3)$

Estimating Probabilities

Disease a prioris are a function of the population for which the expert system is to be used. This is local knowledge and should be adapted to each new setting if the data are available. If the prevalence of a disease in a given population is unknown, an estimate can be made with reference to some other disease for which a relationship is known or inferred within a given population. For example, if the prevalence of melanoma is known to be about 1/6 of that of primary lung‘ cancer and the prevalence of primary lung cancer in the system is .001, then the prevalence of melanoma can be taken as .00016.

If a disease is a subset of a mutually exclusive set of diseases in which the total prevalence is known, then estimates can be made based on the percent contribution of each. For example, if the prevalence of renal failure is taken as .001 and it is known that acute renal failure accounts for 2/3 of the total, then the prevalence of acute renal failure can be taken as .00067 and that of chronic renal failure as .00033.

Problems may arise in some domains such as infectious disease where cases of a given disease may be sporadic or seasonal. In this case, the prevalence can be taken as the average over the year, and the seasonality is taken into account by another finding within the frame. Diseases that (i) only appear in females, (ii) only appear in certain age groups, or (iii) are geographically distributed are handled in the same way.

Testing Frames in Isolation

If the frame editor has a built-in Bayesian calculator, the incipient frame can be loaded into the calculator at any stage of the development process and subjected to a "what-if analysis". This exercise is frequently helpful to experts, especially in looking at combinations of findings. By comparing the result with an expected outcome, numbers can be revised until the frame performs to the satisfaction of the expert. This "tuning process" permits the expert to see immediately the implications of their initial estimate of sensitivity and specificity and thus provides an important insight into the behavior of the frame in various circumstances.

Sources of Error

There are numerous sources of error in building frames:

- Inaccurate probabilities
- Treating findings as independent that are not, i.e., partial nonindependence
- Incomplete frames
- Inappropriate organization within a frame
- Inappropriate clustering
- Errors of logic

It may be difficult to quantify the relative contributions of each of these possibilities. The general procedure is to consider each source of error separately and try to compare and contrast sensible alternatives, using the expert as the gold standard while entering data from real patients having the disease or diseases in question. Once entered, these data are stored for future use in evaluating the knowledge base after changes have been made.

Tools to Facilitate the Knowledge Engineering Process

Text Editor and Database

The initial version of a frame is constructed in a more or less free text format. A frame editor called KESS (knowledge engineering support system) has been developed for the Iliad system that greatly facilitates the construction of these frames and the exchange of information between the knowledge engineer and the expert(s). An early version of this editor was described in 1988[33] that incorporated some concepts originally proposed by Ben Said[51] and some new ideas. Similar tools have been developed and described for other expert systems.[29,52] Users of this book may wish to construct their own frame editor using currently available software tools (e.g., Visual Basic/ACCESS, HyperCard, FoxPro). Some useful features of the KESS database application are described next.

A Working Outline or Hierarchy

Having a list of the frames in the knowledge base, both complete and under construction, is very helpful (see Appendix 1). This may be in the form of a simple alphabetical list of frame names or may include hierarchical relationships between the frames. Additional labels and headings may be added to the directory for organizational purposes.

Accessing Normal Values and Frequently Used Numbers

Quick access to frequently used information such as a list of laboratory tests and their normal ranges and age distributions in the population of interest will speed the knowledge engineering process and provide consistency between frames.

Accessing the Dictionary

The existing dictionary can be made available within the editor, so that existing terminology can be used. This will reduce clerical errors and inconsistencies and save retyping of dictionary terms. However, care must be taken that too much of the expert's time is not wasted while mapping concepts he or she wishes to express to terms in the dictionary when the mapping is obvious and does not justify involving the expert. This can slow down or interfere with the dialogue with the expert.

Maintaining Consistency Between Numerical Estimates

An effort should be made to use consistent false positive values for a given finding in different frames. Being able to see what previous estimates were when building new frames will facilitate this objective. For rare disorders used as findings in another frame, a priori values may be used to estimate false positive rates. For example:

Finding	TP	FP
•Multiple endocrine neoplasms, type II	.60	.0000075

"Multiple endocrine neoplasms, type II" is a finding in a frame called "Medullary carcinoma of the thyroid" in Iliad. The prevalence of "Multiple endocrine neoplasms, type II" is taken as .0000075 in this expert system. The false positive rate in the medullary carcinoma frame is the frequency of the finding in the patients who do not have medullary carcinoma. This would be approximately equal to the prevalence of the disease in the population or, more accurately .0000075 × (1 − .60), which subtracts the fraction found in medullary carcinoma.

Relationships Between Frames

A mechanism to hyperlink between parent frames and subframes is very helpful in the knowledge engineering process. This helps the designer keep in mind relationships within the frame hierarchy. Frequently it is desirable to review other frames for comparison purposes to see how things were done in another case. A general search function should also be available. In a large knowledge base with hundreds of clusters designed over a protracted period of time, it may be difficult to remember which clusters have already been constructed and what naming conventions were used. Because there are usually multiple ways of organizing a frame, it is beneficial to be able to quickly refer to closely related frames for comparison purposes.

Documenting Sources of Knowledge and the Knowledge Engineering Process

Documented sources include the patient database, literature (journals, books, etc.), and experts. Sources of information should be documented so that when a frame is updated or being used as a model to build a subsequent frame, the source and confidence in the source of the information can be determined. If new information from another source is to be merged with existing data, knowing the source of the original data can be a help in deciding how to weigh both sources in the merging process. In some cases, it becomes desirable to make a frame more robust at a later date. If the original references are recorded, they can quickly be accessed for additional information. In some cases, a frame will behave unexpectedly during the testing phase. When the problem can be traced to certain numbers in the frame, it is helpful to be able to determine the source and certainty of those numbers. It is also advisable to record the reasoning used in making estimates, if it is not obvious. Additional notes about mechanisms and future plans may be helpful. Some examples are given below:

Notes about knowledge engineering
•Sepsis
  We took fever, tachycardia, and tachypnea out of this frame, because we are

assuming that information is coming through the septic shock cluster by partial information.

Clinical definitions
•Clinically significant diarrhea
The diarrhea is clinically significant if it is truly present and if there is either intestinal bleeding or signs of infection or tenderness.

•Cystic hygroma
Definition: a multiloculated cystic structure containing lymphatic fluid that is of congenital origin, usually found at the root of the neck and the upper mediastinum or upper thorax.

Notes about estimating a prioris and other probabilities
•Choledocholithiasis
7% of patients with symptomatic gallbladder disease have stones; virtually all these have chronic cholecystitis. About 3/day at LDS Hospital or .003 have an operation for gallbladder disease; 7% of that is .00021.

•Gastroschisis
1/4000 newborns have open abdominal wall defects, and gastroschisis represents about 2/3 of these; the other 1/3 are omphalocele.

•Cystic fibrosis
CF occurs in 1/2500 live births in caucasians; many die in childhood. Most are diagnosed in childhood, but some mild cases are not. Median survival is 25 years. There are probably about 1/year of adult CF in our hospital (20,000 inpatients/year); 1/20,000 = .00005.

•Alpha-1-antitrypsin deficiency emphysema
The gene frequency 0.0122 and the homozygous frequency is .00015, but only 3/4 of these get the disease, so the a priori is .00011. About 3% of all emphysema is caused by AAT deficiency.

Notes about methods
•Arteriosclerosis obliterans (peripheral vascular disease)
Angiography identifies irregularity in the vessel wall with sites of stenosis or obstruction, and it also identifies distal arterial refill and patency in the distal runoff.
Duplex scan with color flow ultrasound shows peripheral arterial disease and blood flow characteristics at various levels in the arterial tree.

Notes about etiology, mechanisms, and clinical presentation
•Lymphedema
The main job of the lymphatics is to pick up proteins. Proteins that leak out of blood vessels are not recovered properly when there is a deficiency of the lymphatic channels. Excess proteins cause accumulation of fluid from oncotic pressure. The protein in the interstices stimulates a fibrotic reaction that gives a ligneus quality to the edema.

•Bartter's syndrome
Renin production with angiotensin insensitivity occurs in this syndrome. The main problem is probably inadequate chloride reabsorption in the ascending loop.

This condition is simulated by situations with decreased K^+ such as covert diuretics and vomiting (with associated K^+ and Mg^{2+} loss)

- Cystinosis
The disease varies in severity from the severe infantile form to a benign form in which retinopathy and renal failure do not occur (patients still have corneal and bone marrow cystine crystals). We are considering the infantile form here.

- Inhalation anthrax
Early symptoms and signs may be very nonspecific (i.e., fever, chest pain, malaise).
Patient status deteriorates very rapidly after 48 to 72 hours depending on the inhaled dose of agent
Inhalation anthrax is not primarily a parenchymal lung disease: spores are carried to mediastinal nodes by pulmonary macrophages where they vegetate and start to produce several toxins. Therefore, although severe dyspnea does occur as a late finding, it is primarily associated with the severe mediastinitis that occurs; the lung fields are generally clear on CXR with the primary CXR findings being widening of the mediastinum and possibly prominence of the hilar nodes.

Saving, Printing, and Statistics

Having the text editor combined with or attached to or part of a database is highly desirable. During the knowledge engineering process, it is frequently necessary to save or print individual frames or sets of frames. When frames are under construction, it is useful to be able to label parts that have changed in a given session so the changes can then be made in the precompiled and compiled versions of the frames (see following). It is then desirable to save or print only the frames that have been modified. To retrieve frames of interest, the user should be able to specify criteria such as medical specialty, date completed, date last updated, partially completed frames, frames with associated treatments, Bayesian or Boolean frames only, final diagnoses only, frames with prevalence <.001, etc. If the frame authoring tool contains separate fields for a priori, specialty, final diagnosis, stage of completion, etc., then such reports can be retrieved by standard searching algorithms.

Combining Frames into a Working System

Mapping Free Text to a Structured Vocabulary

The initial design of the dictionary should be done with much thought and great care. The organization of the dictionary affects data entry, appearance of data in the patient history window, and the speed and accuracy of the inferencing process.

The dictionary should be well organized, comprehensive, and nonredundant (see Chapter 4). Consistency should be maintained at all levels in such aspects as the phrasing of terms, the organization of subhierarchies, and the use of keywords.

By introducing another layer between the dictionary and the user and/or the frames, it is possible to have a single finding in multiple places in the dictionary. Some subsetting can be done by keywording in the dictionary, but this does not facilitate data entry or data presentation in multiple templates.

In many specialties, there is more than one way to organize a section of the dictionary. Decisions can be made based on organizational principles intrinsic to the dictionary or can be guided by the way the terms will be used in practice. For example, patients may complain of pain, stiffness, or swelling of any joint. Should the dictionary be organized as

---

Musculoskeletal symptoms:
  Hx of joint pain
    in the shoulder
    in the wrist
    . . .
  Hx of joint swelling
    in the shoulder
    in the wrist
    . . .
  Hx of joint stiffness
    in the shoulder
    in the wrist
    . . .

Or should the dictionary be organized as

Musculoskeletal symptoms:
  Hx of shoulder complaint(s)
    pain
    stiffness
    swelling
  Hx of wrist complaint(s)
    pain
    stiffness
    swelling

The second organization probably better represents the way the data are obtained from the patient in actual practice.

There are challenging problems of matching data dictionary structure and organization to fit the needs for data input and for decision making.

One goal is to separate the concept from the context to prevent duplication of concepts for each context (i.e., simplify the dictionary) and, more importantly, recognize a concept as the same in multiple contexts (i.e., simplify the knowledge base). It then becomes possible to include the same finding as a member of multiple sets, e.g., serum sodium may be a part of chem7, chem20, chem27; serum cholesterol may be a part of chem20 and a lipid profile. This requires a new table for use with data entry that will allow the user to choose in which contexts a given concept might be expressed.

Another goal is to handle concept modifiers without having to replicate them with each concept they modify, e.g., right/left, acute/chronic. Building a data structure that allows a concept to be linked dynamically to any appropriate modifier (so-called wild-card modifiers) simplifies the dictionary. The trade-off is that this construct may not allow all appropriate modifiers for a given concept to be presented to the user during data entry (as is possible when the modifiers are represented as part of the individual concept hierarchies). These data structures might be unique to each context because the concept modifiers also are context dependent; e.g., time modifiers are appropriate in the context of a patient history of a lump in the breast, but not in the context of a lump found on physical examination of the patient. Such data structures have been described in the literature.[53]

Compiling Frames into a Working Knowledge Base

A software tool is needed to map selected dictionary terms to a precompiled version of each frame. These frames then need to be compiled into a form that can be executed by the inference engine as efficiently as possible. Because in the initial version of the frame the data items (findings) are expressed in free text, mapping these text expressions to items in the structured dictionary usually requires some human intervention to resolve ambiguities that are encountered (see frame authoring, Chapter 9). When the compilation is complete, the expert system is ready to run with the new or modified frames.

6
Evaluation of the Model

Testing and Refining the Compiled Knowledge

In the evaluation phase, the expert system is tested by comparing the differential diagnosis at each stage of the patient workup with the expert's opinion and determining where the knowledge base might be revised to improve performance. This process is carried out first. If the system appears to be overconfident about a particular diagnosis (i.e., assigns a higher probability to that diagnosis than the expert thinks appropriate), suspicion is raised that the false positive rate assigned to some data item already entered for the patient being diagnosed is too low. Another explanation might be that highly associated findings are being treated as independent; i.e., they need to be represented as an "or" group or built into a cluster.

After a new frame has been integrated into the rest of the knowledge base, the expert may judge, after a few findings have been entered, whether the posterior probability of the new frame is appropriate with respect to other diseases listed on the differential. Other program options in Iliad can also help in the evaluation at this stage. The "minimal diagnosis" option that finds the most likely diagnosis which explains the largest number of the patient's abnormal findings is particularly useful. Running this option removes all findings for the disease selected and then forms a new differential based on the unexplained findings. This is a good way for the expert to discover findings that should have been included in the frame but were overlooked.

Appropriateness of Decisions Based on Data Entered by Experts

Entering a few items of data may not be a fair test of the system. In practice, the patient may fill out a form or be questioned by a nurse, which would provide some basic present, past, and family history. The patient would then be examined and various tests ordered with the results available at some later time. One method of data entry for testing the system is to enter all the data (with or without the sine qua non data) at once from a patient's chart or from a transcription record. However, *the most useful role of an expert system is to assist the diagnostic process at intermediate stages*, not after the results of the biopsy are available. Consequently, frames should be tested at each stage of the workup, i.e., after entry of symptoms, signs, lab test, imaging, and special test results. Also, various combinations of findings that could be conceived to be clinically relevant can be entered. It is sometimes possible to "trick" an expert system by giving some set of findings that would be expected to put the disease on the differential list but which fails to do so. It is often the case in these instances that the presentation is unrealistic. In other words, the tests entered would not have been performed in practice without some additional suggestive data.

Testing with Data Newly Entered from Patient Charts

Patient charts usually have incomplete data, and some of these are in a different form than that used by the system. Thus, the data have to be extracted and filtered by a clinician. Some charts are so incomplete as not to be useful. Larger numbers of cases and more varied presentations facilitate the validation process. Simple straightforward cases are useful but not adequate. Some patients are so complicated, with many coexisting diseases in various stages of progression, that they do not provide good test data. On the other hand, real patients do have multiple diseases and the system should be able to sort these out in most cases. Published CPC (clinicopathologic conference) cases are a common source of useful data, but they are usually very incomplete and atypical.

Testing with Cases Stored Earlier

A series of test cases can be accumulated. These cases can be reopened after changes are made to the frames or to the software to see the effects of the changes. They can also be used for various educational purposes, e.g., turned into simulations (see following) that can be worked up by medical students, nursing students, and physician assistants. For this purpose, it is desirable to store vignettes at various stages of completion.

Modifying Source Frames As Required: The Iterative Process

When problems are found during testing, changes are made in the frame editor environment. Having the program and the frame editor open simultaneously facilitates the iterative process of testing, changing, and retesting. During the testing process, it may be apparent that a frame is overconfident, i.e., it comes up too high on the differential or is difficult to get off the differential. This behavior may result from inaccurately estimating too high of an a priori or from inappropriate TP/FP ratios. It may be necessary to reorganize findings within a frame, to combine findings in "or groups" or to include significant negative findings.

7
Applications of the Model

Modes of Use

A medical expert system can be designed to support various modes of use, e.g., consulting mode, critiquing mode, simulation mode, or testing mode.

Consultation Mode

The consultation mode in Iliad is the most common mode of use. The user simply enters the patient data using keywords or a hierarchical data entry. Iliad presents an organized list of structured (i.e., consistent with the hierarchical organization of the dictionary) data elements from the data dictionary, which correspond to the keywords entered by the user. The user answers the questions: yes, no, unknown; or ignores them. A differential diagnostic list is then generated. At this point the user can select a disease from the differential and browse the corresponding frame. Findings can be entered or edited from within the frame. Additional findings can be entered using another set of keywords at any time.

Another option ("best information") is to let Iliad request the most pertinent information pertaining to the top five diseases on the differential. Iliad can also select the disease that accounts for the most findings, subtract those findings from the patient data window, and create a new differential (the "minimal diagnosis" option). The user can request treatment recommendations for diseases on the differential. In addition, some findings in the patient data window are linked to digitized pictures.

Critiquing Mode

When the clinician suspects the patient has a specific disease, the hypothesis can be critiqued by the expert system.[54] This mode greatly simplifies the data entry process because it filters only those questions that are necessary to determine the presence or absence of the disease in question. Numerous other filters can be imagined to restrict data entry. It is possible to access the full dictionary of findings if it becomes necessary while in the critiquing mode.

Simulation Mode

A medical expert system such as Iliad has the capability of presenting simulated cases. In running a simulation, the user requests the answers (values) for any of Iliad's findings for a given case. Requesting data in a simulation is equivalent to entering data in a consult. After each finding is added, the differential and patient history list are updated.

Realistic simulations are best constructed starting with real cases or typical cases. Cases that have been entered in the consulting mode can be automatically converted to simulations. These cases are also useful for evaluating the system. Additional preparation is necessary to make useful simulations. For example, if the user asks for the result of a certain finding that was not part of the case, Iliad will inform the user that it is negative. In many cases, it would be better to inform the user that the data are unknown. However, in some cases the data should not be unknown but the designer of the simulation may have forgotten to add it. In general, all the findings in the frame being simulated (and in closely competing frames) should have answers (i.e., values). Also, if diagnostic data can be supplied by various methods, all the results should be consistent. For example, if there is a liver mass observable by flat plate x-ray, it would probably also be observable by ultrasound and by MRI. Consequently, the designer of the simulation should enter consistent answers for all methods that could be used to get the data (because they could be potentially requested by the user).

The simulation mode may also have an associated scoring algorithm[55] to monitor the user's performance and a "testing mode" in which the user runs a simulation without being able to get any of the normal feedback available within the system. The Iliad simulator has been used at the University of Utah School of Medicine for 5 years[56-58] and at some other medical schools.

The User Interface

No matter how good an expert system is in terms of accuracy, reliability, robustness, etc., how and if it will be used is critically dependent on the user interface. The user interface facilitates data input, browsing, editing, and output.

The available options of the software should be rich enough to satisfy the most sophisticated users, yet organized in such a way that basic features can be easily learned and used by new or unsophisticated users. Related features should be accessible through a common menu, picklist, tool palette, etc. Wherever possible, features should be available via both the keyboard and the mouse.

Input

Input of data is arguably the most critical part of the user interface because it determines the communication between the user and the application. The user needs to enter data and search for information contained in the knowlege base or the database. The ability to enter data will be limited by the robustness and organization of the structured dictionary because only dictionary terms are recognized by the program. The user has to match their query to those terms. This usually involves keyword entry or selecting from picklists. Picklists are useful if they are well organized and not too large. The order of the displayed list should not be dependent on some arbitrary organization within the dictionary. Ideally, the picklists should be tailored to the specific audience (e.g., patient or medication list for clinics or individual physicians) and possibly be customizeable by the user. Example picklists for symptoms that are fairly domain specific can be found in Appendix 4.

Data entry may be the biggest barrier to the use of a medical expert system. In general, if designed properly, the system will perform better with more information and more specific information. However, more information generally equates to more time and effort on the part of the user. The system will not be used efficiently, especially by physicians, if it requires significant time and effort. In this case, physicians may be willing to use it only for occasional cases of special interest. Various methods of reducing this problem can be imagined and attempted, e.g., direct data entry from a patient database, partial data entry by other personnel, use of scanned documents, and direct voice entry.

Some applications make use of predesigned filters and templates that correspond to familiar paper-based forms, e.g., the electronic equivalents of lab slips for chemistry, hematology, and microbiology. Another approach is context-based or event definition[59] data entry (see Chapter 4).

Iliad makes use of inferencing within the dictionary (see Chapter 4 and following) and data relations to improve the rate and amount of data entered. The ability to say yes or no at the cluster level without documenting the finding can speed up data entry in Iliad. Such "complex finding" clusters are labeled as being inferred {Inf} to differentiate them from documented clusters. Subesequent entry of component findings within the cluster will override nondocumented data entry.

Output

Users can save or print individual windows within Iliad or various parts of a case at any stage during the workup. If an expert system is linked to a patient database (not presently available in Iliad), numerous additional reports can be designed. Statistical algorithms can also be added to make such reports more informative (e.g., mean, standard deviation, coefficient of variation).

Browsing Frames

The user can browse individual frames at any stage during the workup in Iliad. The frame is presented in such a way that the user can easily determine why it has a given posteriori probability. The current values of constituent findings can be displayed. It is possible to hypertext to subsidiary clusters, or to view "or groups," display logic, risk flags, etc. It is also possible to input or edit data while browsing the frame.

Viewing and Using the Differential

The differential list in Iliad can be viewed as a single probability-ordered list of top-level diagnoses or as an expanded list showing constituent clusters. A popup list of frame-specific options such as "add data," "explain findings," or "show treatment suggestions" is very convenient. Another useful feature is an option to simultaneously see the current posteriori probability of each frame on the list and the previous probability before inputting data. It would also be useful (although not presently available) to be able to select multiple diagnoses simultaneously, then to ask for "most useful information" (see following) in the context of this subset of diseases.

Patient Data Window

The patient data window displays a list of the data that have currently been entered for a given patient. The information is structured by marking abnormal findings with bold (color coding would also be nice) to show hierarchical relationships. Different types of data (i.e., symptoms, signs, labs, etc.) are separated under appropriate headings. Selecting a given finding (or findings) allows the user to edit, link to pictures, or "explain findings."

Explain Findings

By selecting a finding on the patient history window, the user is able to get a list of all the diseases currently on the differential or all the diseases in the system which use that finding. It would also be useful to be able to select multiple findings and ask the same questions.

Most Useful Information

Iliad will offer suggestions for the next best information to obtain at any stage of the patient workup.[55] These suggestions are based on the information content (see Chapter 3) of the top five diagnoses on the differential list. These suggestions can be limited to history, PE, or lab. It would also be useful to select multiple diagnoses and then to get suggestions as to the best questions or tests that would differentiate, rule in, or rule out those disorders. "Most useful information" includes the cost of acquiring some information. However, it is difficult to assign costs to signs and symptoms as well as complex findings. It should be clear whether designated costs include the physician's cost. Ideally, costs should be kept up to date and modified according to geographic location.

Minimal Diagnosis

In the real world, patients may have multiple diseases simultaneously. The status of diseases can be acute, chronic, intermittent, active/inactive/in remission, etc. Also, because some findings are common to many diseases, it is useful to be able to ask the computer "Which disease explains the most findings?"; this is the essence of the minimal diagnosis algorithm. It is then useful to see what findings are left unexplained on the patient history list. This process can be repeated with the remaining findings.

Bayes Calculator

Because the Iliad expert system is based on a sequential Bayesian model, it is useful to look at individual frames in isolation and to essentially do a "what if analysis." While browsing a frame, the user can "dump" the current patient data into a Bayesian calculator where various combinations of findings can be tested. The user can even select clusters within a frame to open another calculator for that frame; the results of that calculation are carried back to the parent frame. The ability to modify the sensitivities, specificities, and prevalences themselves enhances the value of this tool.

Interfaces to Other Knowledge

Numerous types of ancillary information are potentially useful during the patient workup and can be linked to the expert system. Under ideal circumstances, any relevant patient-specific information would be at the caregiver's fingertips. Besides a working differential diagnostic list, this would include previous patient data and images and treatment suggestions. Secondary information would include definitions of clinical terms, drug information, literature reports of treatment options, ICD9[60] or CPT[61] codes, insurance information, etc. The main difference between accessing this information from a database and from an expert system is that some "intelligence" can be built into the system so that the information retrieved is more meaningful or expedient. Drug alerts can be generated, for example, by comparing a patient's drug orders, lab data, etc. with a table of known drug interactions. Note that these suggestions are patient- and time specific.

Relevant Literature

A tremendous amount of basic research goes on worldwide; some percentage of this is clinically related. This literature may pertain to etiology, medical genetics, pathological mechanisms, diagnostic evaluation and methodology, treatment methods, management protocols, prognosis, and quality and cost of medical care. No practicing clinician can hope to keep up on more than a small percentage of the literature at this level. Numerous medical groups and organizations review and filter this information, thereby producing summary reports and recommendations. These recommendations may form the basis of some clinical trials, which may then lead to some level of validation of some of these recommendations for certain conditions, disorders, or patients. Reports of these validated studies may be reported in certain prestigious journals, medical textbooks, conferences, etc. Some of this information will reach practicing physicians who may take advantage of it; others will continue to practice medicine in ignorance of new and potentially important information. What is needed is some means of making the pertinent information available to the clinician precisely at the time it may be potentially useful for a given patient and circumstance. A properly designed and connected medical expert system has that potential.

Pictures

Radiological images (e.g., plain film x-rays, CT, MRI, ultrasound, endoscopy, echocardiograms, nuclear imaging) are a central part of medical care. All these images can now be digitized and stored in a central database, from which they can be instantly retrieved. Digitized photographic images of gross pathological specimens, skin lesions, etc., are very useful in diagnosis and treatment of some diseases. Within an expert system, images can be linked to specific findings and disease names.[62] Ideally, the user should be able to bring up sample images for comparison of similar lesions (or the same kinds of lesions differing in severity or presentation) by typing in appropriate keywords or selecting from picklists. Presenting multiple images first as "thumbnails" from which the user can select and enlarge is very useful. The ability to select images or portions of images to zoom in, copy, crop, or print is also desirable.

Sound

Heart, chest, and bowel sounds can be stored digitally. Conceiveably, some decision support system could assist a user in interpreting sounds recorded during the physical exam of a patient (analogous to ECG interpretation, which has been in place for many years[63]).

Animation/Video

Short animations of proper methods for doing physical exams would be useful to many clinicians, e.g., proper methods for doing musculoskeletal, motor, sensory, or thyroid exam. Videos of patients with various kinds of tics, tremors, or gait abnormalities could be linked to an expert system. Graphical comparisons of the advantages and disadvantages of different potential treatments would also be helpful.

ICD9 Codes

Being able to select a disease name in the application and request the ICD9 code is a useful option for practicing physicians. Undoubtedly this will not be a one-to-one mapping. In some cases there will be more than one ICD9 code and vice versa. In other cases there will be no corresponding ICD9 code because names and definitions of diseases in the expert system may differ from those in ICD9.

Other Coding Systems

Being able to load patient data directly from various sources could greatly increase the potential value of an expert system. This would require translation tables or a "vocabulary server"[49] that could map the patient's data into terms the expert system understands.

Other Expert Systems

Taking another quantum leap, once expert systems become generally available and thoroughly validated, it will become apparent that each system has strengths and weaknesses. It will then be useful to be able to transfer information between expert systems. Some effort has been made in recent years to exchange decision support tools, e.g., medical logic modules.[64]

Compromises

Ease of Data Entry Versus Confusion Regarding "Inferred No"

The "inferred no" (see Chapter 4) is a construct designed mainly to facilitate data entry and generate a more realistic differential. The basic assumption is that, if the user has entered data from a part of the dictionary hierarchy, it is safe to assume that all associated items were not present, because they would presumably also have been entered. If an "inferred no" flag is used in a subhierarchy of the dictionary, it must be set at the appropriate level, so as to be relatively certain that the user would have seen all the associated data. This may vary with the user and the mode of entry. In any case, the user must be aware of this construct and the data must be duly recorded in the patient window. There may be times when the user wants to use the "inferred no" and others when it is undesirable. Perhaps an "all others no" button would be more appropriate or, possibly, the "inferred no" could be associated with data entry filters or templates.

Response Time Versus Sophistication of Algorithm

The Iliad expert system has about 3100 frames and 15,000 findings. When large amounts of data are entered simultaneously, it is necessary to process each finding through every frame that uses it, followed by processing each of these frames through every frame which uses that frame as a complex finding. Yes and no inferencing within the dictionary, the "inferred no," and data relations (see Chapter 4) can greatly increase the number of findings that need to be processed simultaneously. Nesting of frames (which may be more than 50 levels in extreme cases) further increases processing time. Incredibly enough, with existing hardware and standard implementations, the user is rarely required to wait more than 1 or 2 seconds. This is largely because Iliad is RAM based, requiring at least 3 MBytes of memory. There are also various performance heuristics, such as (i) if only negative findings are present, do not process the frame; (ii) if only a double negative is present, do not process the frame; (iii) if only risk flags are present, do not process the frame. Empirically it can be shown that there is very little effect on calculations when more than three levels of nesting are considered in most cases. Other heuristics could be adopted, such as "If the effect of the calculation would affect the posteriori probability of the frame by <1%, do not process the finding at the present time."

Attempts have been made in Iliad to limit the levels of nesting, both for performance reasons and because it seems inconsistent with the way clinicians diagnose diseases. It also makes it difficult to backtrack and determine why certain findings have a given effect on diseases of interest. One attempt to diminish the "infinite nesting" problem was to limit all "risk frames" to one level of depth. There were many "At risk for . . ." frames in Iliad that contained a list of predisposing diagnoses; e.g., "At risk for chronic renal failure" included "Diabetic nephropathy," which included "NIDDM," which included "At risk for NIDDM," etc.:

Chronic renal failure
- At risk for chronic renal failure
- Diabetic nephropathy
- NIDDM
- At risk for NIDDM

The reasoning behind this was as follows: as findings for NIDDM were entered, the probability of NIDDM would increase, which would then increase the likelihood of diabetic nephropathy (if there were any associated nephropathy), which would pass information to the "At risk for chronic renal failure" frame, which would then drive the "Chronic renal failure" frame. When all the disorders listed in "At risk for chronic renal failure" were changed to "Hx of . . ." or "Past Hx of . . .", this meant that information would not automatically be passed when the probability of NIDDM increased. "At risk for chronic renal failure" will only be driven if the user enters "Hx of NIDDM." Conceivably, some relationship could be algorithmically formulated between "Hx of NIDDM" and the "NIDDM" frame.

Once it becomes possible to represent a disease simultaneously as a disease frame, a "Hx of . . ." and a "Past Hx of . . .", an ambiguity is immediately introduced both in terms of data entry and in terms of data representation within the expert system. In addition, there is a potential "infinite loop" problem. There are some diseases that may be diagnosed either before or after the diagnosis of an associated disease; e.g., patients with "Pulmonary embolus" are at risk for "Deep venous thrombophlebitis" and vice versa. Should the frame "Pulmonary embolus" contain the finding "Deep venous thrombophlebitis" and the frame "Deep venous thrombophlebitis" contain the finding "pulmonary embolus," a potential "infinite loop" would be created (with one frame calling another frame, which then calls the original frame). Perhaps "Pulmonary embolus" should include "Hx of DVT" or "Past Hx of DVT" or "At risk for DVT." Would there be any advantage in including all these possibilities with different sensitivities and specificities? Would it make more sense to have some inherent relationship between them? Whatever the decision, it should be done consistently throughout the expert system. Such decisions can have a large effect on performance.

Our limited experience with Bayesian networks suggests that attempting to relate all findings to each other increases the processing time by at least an order of magnitude for a large expert system.[22] Neural net models[65] would be expected to have similar performance penalties. However, it is conceivable that advantages such as improved performance could outweigh disadvantages in a small knowledge base or when implemented in a "high-powered" environment, if all the requisite parameters could somehow be ascertained.

Once the expert system is linked to a patient database, searching within the patient database may become more of a limiting factor. This problem could be minimized if the expert system essentially runs in the background or intermediate results are stored or cached.

8
Lessons Learned

Teaching Medical Clerks, Physician Assistants, and Other Trainees

Iliad was initially developed as a tool for use by third-year medical students at the University of Utah during their clerkship on the internal medicine wards.[56-58] It was intended to facilitate the learning that occurs during the student's first real contact with patients. Four specific goals influenced the design of this expert system.

The first goal was to provide, through Iliad, a source of consultation to the student during the diagnostic workup of a patient. The use of the consultation mode by medical students has provided help in working up cases for presentation on rounds where the student is expected to provide a differential diagnosis, given some or all of a patient's findings. In this mode some students have also found the best information algorithm useful in suggesting appropriate information to gather during the workup of a patient.

The second goal was to provide experience with a much broader set of diseases than could possibly be provided to the student with the limits on number and variety of patients seen on the inpatient wards of a teaching hospital. This, of course, is provided using the simulation mode. All students were required to solve at least two simulated cases each week of the 12-week medicine clerkship. Many students solved many times this number, exploring cases from all the specialties of internal medicine.

The third goal was to provide convenient and sophisticated computer-based tools for browsing the features of diseases such as incidence, disease manifestations, and risk factors. Students use this browse function to find the relationships between findings and diseases that often involve multiple levels of reasoning and explain these relationships in terms of the pathophysiological processes involved. Knowledge of these processes can then be used to reason clinically instead of relying on memorization of a list of possible findings to look for in a patient suspected of having a given disease. Early versions of Iliad, which linked each disease name to a selected subset of recent medical literature abstracts, provided some students with a convenient entry point for accessing relevant material for rounds with residents and faculty.

A fourth goal was to introduce the student to concepts involved in making treatment decisions once a diagnosis has been established. In spite of the emphasis on learning diagnosis in the third-year medicine clerkship, students also participate in discussions of treatment. Iliad provides enough knowledge about treatment options for each disease to give the student a foundation for understanding some of the treatment issues being discussed on rounds.

Medical students at the University of Utah are trained to use Iliad during their first week on the medicine clerkship in a computer lab at the medical library. Training is done in groups of 10 in a training room equipped with a workstation for each student and takes 3 hours to complete. After a brief description of the program, each student follows the demonstration of Iliad (used in the consultation mode) by going through each step of a workup and trying each of the system's options on their own computer. The students then explore the program on their own with the instructor available to answer questions. This sequence is then repeated using the simulation mode. At the end of the training session, the instructor outlines the clerkship requirements in terms of cases to be solved and tests to be given each week. Each students is assigned to one of the workstations in place on the wards of one of the three teaching hospitals.

As students perform simulated and test cases throughout their internal medicine rotation, Iliad evaluates each user's performance against its own and assigns a performance score. This score represents a measure of the user's ability to interpret the data available and generate probable hypotheses. During the past several years, analysis of the scores of the students suggests that students performing Iliad simulation cases diagnose more accurately at a lower cost than those who are not trained with Iliad.[47]

Iliad is being tried in many situations other than on the wards with third-year medical students. As a teaching tool, Iliad is also being used routinely by student physician assistants and nurse practitioners. Both these groups have enthusiastically adopted Iliad as an integral part of their curriculum and have little trouble using the program effectively after experiencing a training session similar to that used to train new medical clerks.

As a teaching tool, Iliad has been used (in some way) in more than half of the medical schools in the United States. In our experience, the support of the faculty and the administration, the preparatory orientation sessions to introduce Iliad to the students, the availability of computers on the patient wards, and the weekly rounds of the technical staff are essential for a successful implementation of such an expert system as part of a medical school curriculum.

As a Tool for Preauthorization

There are several other areas where an expert diagnostic system might prove useful and in which we have already had some experience. In the setting of a health maintenance organization, an expert diagnostic system has proved useful as an objective tool for preauthorization of planned diagnostic or surgical procedures.

Using Iliad knowledge engineering tools, a special knowledge base was developed to describe the indications for surgery (IliadPro). The most frequently performed surgeries were identified, and a first draft of the indications for each surgery was defined by one domain expert. The initial knowledge base was then reviewed by a panel of experts from each surgical specialty, and modifications were made until a consensus was reached. The final knowledge base was implemented at a health insurance preauthorization service. For each surgery, a form listing the data necessary to evaluate the indications for that surgery was distributed to the participating surgeons. The forms were filled out and faxed to the preauthorization nurse, who entered the data into the IliadPro system. The program then generated an approval or a referral decision with detailed explanations in both situations.[65]

The knowledge engineering for this kind of task should involve enough physicians who are actually engaged in making these decisions in their own practice so that the criteria developed will indeed represent a consensus that all the physicians can accept in their everyday practice. Another lesson learned is that although experts acknowledged the "guidelines" in practice, their own cases were rejected by the system for lack of documentation or deviation from guidelines.

One clear benefit of the computerized preauthorization system was to provide an objective level of documentation for the reasons for surgery. Also, integration of this tool with the medical record would enhance its direct use by the provider.

As a Screening Tool for Quality Improvement

Another way a diagnostic expert system has been used to advantage is monitoring the quality of health care using patient charts. The standard practice in the United States usually involves nurses reviewing a random selection of charts using a protocol with rules to define deviations from accepted practice. The primary focus of this kind of review is detection of procedural errors such as failure to sign an operative permit or missing documentation. A very large fraction of errors flagged by the nurse review were not considered clinically significant when reviewed by an expert panel, and errors in diagnosis were not even searched. An experiment was performed using Iliad to detect diagnostic errors in these charts by having nurses enter data from the chart and then looking for differences in the attending physicians diagnoses and Iliad's differential.[67] Significant clinical errors were detected using this approach, and they were different than the errors found by the standard protocol.

Commercial Users of Iliad

There are several thousand individual users of Iliad. A recent survey yielded the following representative responses from this group:

Positive experiences:
    Iliad has helped generate some useful DDx's and helped confirm suspicious or complicated cases.
    In consultation, Iliad suggested primary and secondary adrenal insufficiency in a patient with nausea, vomiting, and vague abdominal pain. Several tests have supported secondary AI. Some tests are still out, but it reminded us of this less common Dx.
    Once it brought up a higher probability of a diagnosis I had not previously considered, suggesting to me to consider it more seriously.
    It is useful in narrowing down the differential diagnosis of renovascular hypertension.
    It ruled out unusual causes of back pain.
    It helps define what tests to order for nonroutine disorders.
    Iliad saved a surgery for possible appendicitis by suggesting the diagnosis could be mononucleosis, and it turned out that was what the patient had.
    It is useful in the sense of developing a complete differential diagnosis list and exhaustively ruling out various possibilities.
    It helps in multiple problem patients.
    It helps to look for something I had overlooked.
    I tested Iliad with 10 internal medicine cases from the archives. Once we mastered the detailed entering of information, the results were (surprisingly) accurate. Especially in some dubious, complex cases, Iliad got on the right track.

Negative experiences:
    I have attempted to use Iliad at the bedside but it is cumbersome.
    I am disappointed in its performance "at the bedside." I practice Emergency Medicine and it requires too much data entry to develop a differential diagnosis list.
    Most of the stuff I look up it does not have info on.
    More instructional than practical.
    Iliad has not prompted me to handle patients any differently yet. I like the likelihood ratios.

I do not use it in a patient's presence. It always confirms my diagnoses
or is just as confused as I.

The problems with Iliad as a consultation tool most frequently cited were
these:

The amount of time required to enter data

The lack of integration of Iliad with the patient information system

The incompleteness of the knowledge base

The irrelevancies in the differential that Iliad can sometimes produce

In response to these problems, a client/server version of Iliad is being
developed that will be able to link with existing computerized patient
records. This link will reduce the data entry time for the user as patient data
can be retrieved automatically from the medical record, given that the host
vocabulary can be translated into Iliad terminology. In addition, ongoing
knowledge engineering efforts are continuously adding and validating the
content and the accuracy of the knowledge base.

9
Knowledge Engineering Tools

Knowledge engineering (KE) tools (i.e., software applications defined for a specific purpose) facilitate a quick cycle time from acquiring information from domain experts, the literature, and patient databases, to restructuring that information in the system and testing its performance against expert judgment and real cases. The process of developing a working knowledge base is iterative, and multiple cycles are necessary before a satisfactory behavior evolves.

Knowledge Acquisition

For the development of the Iliad expert system, domain experts and knowledge engineers meet to define new frames or test existing ones on a weekly basis. A special room and seating arrangement have been used to facilitate this process. A glass-topped table is supported by four supports housing computer monitors set at an angle to optimize viewing; the monitors are connected on a common network and can be switched to display output from computers on either end of the table. Participants in the engineering process can interact with good eye contact while referring to the same information on the visual displays underneath the table. Various other equivalent arrangements could be imagined.

A database application called KESS (knowledge engineering support system) was developed (see Chapter 5). KESS contains a directory of all the frames in Iliad with individual records for each frame. The hierarchical directories (see Appendix 1) are organized by medical specialty. Using hyperlinks in the directory and the individual frame records, the user can click on the name of a disease and access the diagnostic and treatment information about that disease. Free text (i.e., noncontrolled) terminolgy is used in KESS in describing diagnostic and treatment information to avoid constraining the dialogue between the domain experts and the knowledge engineers. The dates of creation and of last revision are saved as well as the names of the experts who contributed to the construction of the frame. The literature references and the reasoning used to reach certain conclusions are also recorded.

Another important part of KESS is the Bayesian calculator. New frames or changed frames can be exported from KESS into a utility program, the Bayesian calculator, which allows testing and adjusting of the prevalence, sensitivity, and specificity estimates for accurate performance of the diagnostic logic.

KESS maintains the master copy of the Iliad knowledge base. After each KE session, newly created frames and modified frames are printed from KESS. These documents are used to update the Iliad data files using the Iliad KE tool (provided on the CD and described in Appendix 3). The various components of the KE process are described next.

Structuring and Coding the Knowledge

In a typical interaction with an expert system, the user presents the system with a list of data elements from a specific case and gets advice and recommendations from the program. For the expert system to understand the user's input, the first step is to create a dictionary of all the data elements known to the expert system.

The Dictionary Program

The dictionary program defines in a nonambiguous way all the terms used in the knowledge base by associating each term with a numeric code. The frames then refer to these codes and not to the text. This construct greatly speeds up processing during runtime.

In Iliad, the dictionary contains symptoms, physical examination findings, laboratory tests, diagnostic procedures, and diagnoses names (see Chapter 4). Each entry in the dictionary includes additional attributes such as synonyms, cost, units of measure, and normal values when it is appropriate. Some items have special flags, e.g., risk flag, display flag, and "inferred no" flag. Furthermore, the dictionary program can define relationships between terms. These can be hierarchical and nonhierarchical relationships. Hierarchical relationships describe parent–child relations as in cough and hemoptysis, rash and vesicle, heart diseases and heart attack, analgesic and aspirin. A common way to capture these hierarchical links is to use hierachical codes. In Iliad, the hierarchical code for hemoptysis, for example, is as follows:

1.0.0.0.0.0	Current Hx
1.10.0.0.0.0	Pulmonary symptoms
1.10.15.0.0.0	Cough
1.10.15.2.0.0	Hemoptysis

Iliad uses a six-part code, which was originally modeled after the dictionary underlying the HELP system.[5,28] In some cases, more levels would be desirable. Iliad has some rules regarding the hierarchy, e.g., "nouns (i.e., main concepts) should be at level 3." Unfortunately, these rules are not rigidly maintained, so that it is possible to have nouns at levels 4, 5, or even 6. As a result, the user cannot depend on main concepts being at level 3 and the program cannot make use of this rule to generate picklists, for example.

Hierarchies can be strict or tangled. A strict hierarchy allows only one parent for any given term while a tangled hierarchy allows for multiple parents. For instance, aspirin can be represented under analgesics and under antipyretics; pneumonia can be classified as a pulmonary or an infectious disease. Nonhierarchical relationships can capture additional knowledge about dependencies between elements in the dictionary. For instance, there are observations that are mutually exclusive (e.g., blood types), observations that automatically take the same value (e.g., CHEM7 glucose and CHEM20 glucose), and observations that are not applicable if another observation is made (e.g., pregnancy and male).

Frame Authoring

Initially, the decision frames are written as free-text (i.e., ASCII) documents, but before these documents can be manipulated by the expert system, they have to be structured and the terminology mapped to the dictionary. The frame authoring tool is used for this task. It validates the syntax, logic, and references to the data dictionary. This tool creates a copy of the decision frame that is strictly structured according to the knowledge model.

The frame authoring tool saves a copy of the knowledge base in a binary format that is ready to be checked and compiled into a form which optimizes its processing by the expert sytem.

Syntax Checking and Compilation

The utilities tool checks the syntax of the decision frames for predefined errors. For example, one utility function checks for decision frames that are referenced by other decision frames but that are missing from the knowledge base. Another utility function identifies frames with undefined data elements (i.e., no reference to the dictionary); this may result from not-yet-mapped terms in the decision frame or from terms mapped to nonexisting entries in the dictionary. Once all errors have been corrected, the knowledge base is ready to be compiled.

The compilation process restructures the elements of the knowledge base to optimize the operations of the expert system. For instance, the compilation process will create an index file of all the dictionary terms used by the knowledge base with links from each dictionary term to the list of the decision frames referencing this term. Thus, as a user selects a dictionary term to describe a specific case, the program can quickly retrieve all decision frames relevant to that entry and update their status (i.e., calculate a new likelihood for that diagnosis).

Starting from a large number of frame authoring documents and the dictionary files, the compilation process results in a small set of compact files serving the needs of the expert system (Iliad uses 13 files contained in a folder called "Iliad files'). The expert system is then used to test the compiled knowledge base.

Testing the Knowledge Base

Review of the output of the expert system by domain experts and knowledge engineering provides feedback as to the behavior of the model and suggests modifications to improve the performance (see Chapter 6). Typically, testing starts with short and "classical" cases (i.e., "textbook cases') to validate the essential correctness of the model. Then, more difficult test cases and real cases with or without concurrent diseases are tried. As deficiencies are encountered, the KE team investigates the reasons for the poor performance and identifies possible remedies. These corrections are made directly in the master copy of the knowledge base using the KESS system. At the end of a testing session, all the changes are saved and printed to be incorporated into a new compile of the knowledge base that will be prepared for the next scheduled testing session. The turnaround time between compilations is fairly quick; compilation of the Iliad knowledge base requires 30 minutes on a Quadra 630 with 16 MBytes of RAM. Many testing cycles are needed before a satisfactory behavior of the model evolves.

Summary

In summary, the KE tools support an iterative process of knowledge acquisition, coding and structuring, and testing, where the richness of the test cases determines the robustness of the performance of the expert system. The main functions of the KE tools allow the knowledge engineer to quickly make changes to the knowledge base without changing or recompiling the application that runs it. Familiarity with the domain content and the expert system model equip the knowledge engineer with the required skills to define a variety of situations that test the system's performance and identify the causes of inadequate performance. This is a continuous quality improvement process that never ends and always yields, with practice, a better expert system.

10
Example Knowledge Bases

The Knowledge Engineering Class

The popularity of medical informatics has been on the upswing for a number of years as the role of computers has increased in importance in health care. The Department of Medical Informatics at the University of Utah has taught a graduate level course in Knowledge Engineering for the past 6 years.

The objectives of the Knowledge Engineering class include (1) providing an overview of computer-assisted decision support models; (2) helping students to use and understand Iliad; (3) teaching students about the medical decision-making process; (4) teaching students the process of knowledge engineering (to capture, restructure, and validate the data that will be used in the knowledge base); (5) teaching students to use the "Iliad KE tool" to build their own medical expert systems; and (6) teaching students to use the Iliad program to test the expert system.

The following are some recent examples of the Knowledge Engineering class projects:

Medically related projects:
Acute abdominal pain in the RLQ (Dominik Aronsky, MD)
Empiric therapy for suspected nosocomial infections in the pediatric ICU (Adrienne Randolph MD)
Diagnosing the diseases causing hyponatremia (Marzena Wisniewska)
Diagnosis of primary lung cancers (Liujie Yang)
Determination of the severity of pneumonia and related risk factors given relevant findings and concurrently determining treatment (Rick Bradshaw)
Preauthorization of cataract surgery (Alan Terry)
Oxygen transport and delivery abnormalities (Tom Oniki)
Diagnosis of blister diseases (W. Hsueh-fen Young)

Diagnosis of prostatic diseases (Roberto de Almeida Rocha)
Diagnosis of nosocomial infections in the hospital environment (Beatriz
    Helena de S. C. Rocha)
Indications for coronary arteriography (Jim Caldwell)
Treating pituitary adenomas (Spencer Koehler)
Recognition and treatment of decubitus ulcers (Suzanne Miller)

Some nonmedical projects:
Modeling the MBA admissions process (Jerome D. Wiest)
Admission to nursing school
Rocket fuel diagnostics
Diagnosing computer network problems
Determining the likelihood of petroleum deposits from sampling of dia-
    toms in soil samples

Medical and Pediatric HouseCall

The time and resources required to develop a large knowledge base system
are tremendous. Thus, it is advisable to develop multiple ways to use these
knowledge bases. This section describes HouseCall, a home medical guide
and symptom analysis program based on the knowledge base of Iliad.

Knowledge of preventive measures and home treatment can potentially
reduce the rate and severity of medical problems while reducing unnecessary health care expenditures. Accurate documentation of a patient's complaints and related information facilitates patient/physician communication
and appropriate treatment of the patient's condition. There is evidence that
an informed patient is better able to provide pertinent information about
their condition and is more cooperative with their treatment.[68–70] This is
important, because in the case of prescription medicine, for example, noncompliance generally yields poor outcomes such as prolonged illness, avoid-
able side effects, drug interactions, increased hospitalization, absences from
work, unnecessary use of health care resources, and even death.[71]

Medical HouseCall is a software program that provides family diagnostic
software and a computerized medical encyclopedia. The expert system
knowledge base, which underlies the "Symptoms analysis" option, is derived from the Iliad knowledge base. In addition to symptom analysis and
the medical encyclopedia, Medical HouseCall has information about drug–
drug interactions and a medical record. HouseCall's most unique feature,
compared to other similar applications currently available, is the symptom
analysis.

Symptom Analysis

In the symptom analysis section, the user begins by entering their age and
gender. Then, the user enters their current symptoms by selecting entries

from lists of findings appearing under body part icons. Medical HouseCall then generates a list of possible causes (a differential diagnosis) ranked by order of likelihood and asks the user "follow-up questions a doctor might ask." The diagnoses listed never exceed 70% (a value representing the average contribution of the historical information toward making a diagnosis, according to some studies[72]), as HouseCall only uses historical information (see following). In most situations a physical exam by a physician or lab tests would be required to confirm a diagnosis.

The knowledge base of 1100 diagnoses contains disease descriptions from internal medicine, neurology, dermatology, pediatrics, OB/GYN, psychiatry, sports medicine, and peripheral vascular diseases and is supported by more than 6000 historical findings phrased in lay language.

Deriving HouseCall from Iliad

HouseCall's "symptom analysis" was derived from Iliad. The Iliad expert system inference engine was restructured to serve HouseCall's needs. The Iliad inference engine was isolated from the data dictionary and the user interface so as to link it to HouseCall's dictionary of lay terms and its more "user-friendly" interface. The information in the personal medical record including past medical history, risk factors, family history, etc., can also be used by the inference engine in determining a differential diagnosis. HouseCall's decision frames are also linked to additional related information such as dictionary definitions and drug information.

Several adjustments were made to adapt to consumers the diagnostic module designed for health care professionals using Iliad. First, Iliad uses symptoms, physical exam findings, and lab results while only symptoms and historical information can be entered in HouseCall. To enhance the performance in HouseCall, additional symptoms and a large number of physical examination findings recognized as patient-observed physical findings (e.g., swollen ankle, red eye, swollen lymph nodes) were added. Second, all history findings were translated into consumer language. To translate the vocabulary to patient language, the same principles used in the translation of Iliad to French and German were adopted.[73] For example, dyspnea was replaced with "shortness of breath," polydipsia with "increased thirst," acute myocardial infarction with "heart attack." A term-to-term translation was not always sufficient; many items had to be separated into their component concepts to facilitate understanding. For instance, the question "smoking history in number of pack/years" was split into two questions: smoking history for "number of years" and "number of packs per day." Third, diagnostic probabilities were adjusted to never exceed 70%. Fourth, diagnoses were combined in broader categories when the differentiation is only possible based on physical examination and lab values. For instance,

HouseCall has one meningitis frame, while Iliad has seven meningitis frames.

A new user interface was built using alphabetical lists containing the primary terms, synonyms, and lexical variants. The multiple windows of Iliad's interface were replaced with a "HyperCard"-like interface that quickly provides the consumer a comfortable familiarity with HouseCall features.

The use of Iliad's inference engine by another application suggests other possibilities such as linking Iliad or HouseCall to other clinical information systems with a medical record component. This would provide diagnostic and treatment decision support and guide the documentation of important signs and symptoms.

Knowledge Engineering for HouseCall

The first knowledge engineering task was to develop the list of topics useful to include in HouseCall. Iliad's knowledge base was supplemented by about 250 additional diagnoses. The intention was to appropriately cover the common medical issues of concern to health care consumers. The list of topics was developed starting with Iliad diagnoses, symptoms, tests, etc. and comparing that against several medical textbooks, consumer reports and books, government publications, and existing consumer software. Each topic was then described using a template that addresses consumer concerns.

The Iliad diagnostic criteria and treatment information provided the starting information of each frame. Then, each HouseCall document was reviewed by additional experts. More than 40 domain experts (physicians, nurses, pharmacists, toxicology experts, dieticians) were consulted to review the initial information for accuracy and completeness. The medically reviewed documents were also reviewed by nurses and editors to ensure consistency of style between the different authors and the level of education required to understand the information.

A number of tools were developed to automatically perform the cross-referencing between documents. Each document in HouseCall has a primary name, a list of synonyms, and a list of lexical variants (e.g., word order, plural forms). The text of each document in HouseCall was scanned against these names to provide automatic hypertexting capabilities from multiple terms, which are color coded.

The program was reviewed by several focus groups of non-health care professionals. For the most part, these user groups found no difficulty operating the program. When asked to express in their own words the value of HouseCall, they used terms such as it provides "needed information for sound medical decision making," it provides "information for people that can't afford or have time to run to the doctor for everything," "it makes you feel you have more control over your own health," and "the real value is that it brings the mysterious and intimidating knowledge of medicine down to Earth and into the home, where it can be used by those who need it."

11
Future Challenges

Links to Patient Data: Client/Server Version of Iliad

Although many expert systems or decision support systems have been developed, used, and evaluated to some extent, the full benefits of this advanced computer technology await their wide use in the health care system. Major obstacles (see also Chapter 1) to the wide dissemination of decision support systems exist, e.g.:

Limited dissemination and completeness of electronic medical records
Limited integration of existing sources of data
Limited integration of clinical data with the natural workflow
Lack of a standard vocabulary
Lack of proven decision support systems

Architecture

One approach to integration of current medical expert system technology to existing information systems is an open architecture, which can be defined as a knowledge server with a general vocabulary interface.

Knowledge Server. The knowledge server (KS) can be conceived as an independent (from the patient database) application running on a platform that optimizes its performance. The KS receives knowledge requests (such as "what is the diagnosis for a given case," "what is the best test given a condition") and responds to them appropriately.

An inference engine restructured into a module of a knowledge server and connected to a patient database would minimize the direct data input required of the physician by using coded clinical data already available in computerized medical records (e.g., laboratory results).

Vocabulary Server. A second component necessary to interface the knowledge server to existing sources of data is the Vocabulary Server (VoSer). The VoSer acts as the information broker between the different components of the overall system and the knowledge server. The VoSer facilitates integration and transfer of patient information acquired by different patient care systems. The strategy is to map the vocabularies of existing information systems to an integrated, "meta"-vocabulary structure. This unified representation then facilitates the translation and exchange of data, and, in particular, allows the KS to automatically examine data stored in the medical record and provide real-time decision support.

The VoSer has two parts: the medical concepts or vocabulary terms, and the templates that describe how these vocabulary entries can be combined to represent meaningful compound terms. The VoSer is the underlying language that unifies the representation of all vocabularies and coding schemes used by the system.

The open (or client/server) architecture allows decision rules and other knowledge constructs to automatically examine the data stored in a medical record and provide real-time decision support. The rules can be triggered by storing or modifying information in the medical record (data driven) or by reaching a set time and date (time driven). The rules can also be triggered voluntarily by the user or in a set batch mode to screen all records.

Applications

The possible applications of linking a clinical data repository to a Knowledge Server include the following.

Documentation: a physician-friendly way to document in detail (coded vs. free text) a patient problem into the clinical data repository using disease descriptions in the knowledge base and patient specific data

Guidelines: practice guidelines, alerts, and reminders that can be automatically activated by the data stored in the clinical database, by the physician, or by other sources such as laboratory or pharmacy systems

Diagnosis: automatic review of patient data to provide diagnostic suggestions

Treatment: suggestion of appropriate treatment alternatives for any given diagnosis

Ordering: cost-effective test ordering suggestions based on the available patient information in the clinical database and the knowledge of the expert system

Quality assurance and continuous quality improvement: decision support is also used to gather relevant information and feedback of current practice patterns, such as the rate of C-section per OB/GYN specialist, the average duration of surgery for various types of surgery, and the length of stay in the hospital. This discreet physician-specific feedback has proven by itself to provide quality improvement and cost reduction of health care processes.[74]

Benefits

The direct benefits of integrated medical expert systems are being measured at various institutions in terms of health care quality improvement, cost reduction, and health promotion and education. Health care payment plans will most likely want and need these tools to enhance patient health outcomes (i.e., quality) while helping their physicians achieve a lower per unit cost. The successful implementation and demonstration of an intelligent Knowledge Server with an intersystem Vocabulary Server can be predicted to have several significant impacts:

The nonintrusive knowledge services (e.g., diagnostic support) provided will increase the use of clinical information systems by clinicians, which means that other systems useful to physicians will be in demand (e.g., prescription writing).

Knowledge-based systems will become more in demand by clinicians and administrators.

Knowledge engineering tools and knowledge engineers will become increasingly in demand.

A market of sharable knowledge bases will develop.

Medical vocabulary and intervocabulary issues will be better understood, potentially accelerating the development of a standard national medical vocabulary.

As richer clinical data repositories containing structured medical history are available, systems to conduct outcome research and epidemiologic studies will develop.

Future Directions

The multimembership Bayesian model used by Iliad has certain weaknesses. It may be difficult to include all relevant negative findings in a frame without making it very complex. Even then, findings not accountable to one disease may be attributed to another disease in the same patient. Iliad uses the "minimal diagnosis" algorithm to find a differential diagnosis that will account for all findings in a patient. Bayesean belief networks (see Chapter 1) are a more sophisticated approach to this problem, but experience has shown this approach to require more computer power than is currently available in a clinic setting for a system as large as Iliad. This model may work well for smaller systems, if the relevant probabilities can be obtained.

The structured vocabulary required for diagnostic expert systems presents a major challenge.[53] For the Iliad system, this component is organized hierarchically and has grown directly from terms used by experts who created the knowledge base. This vocabulary starts with basic concepts such as "cough" or "headache" and then adds modifiers at a lower level of the hierarchy to complete the phrase. Providing easy and natural means for a user of Iliad to enter these findings by matching an entered phrase or word is sometimes difficult even with large sets of synonyms available. Allowing the user to specify the context (history of present illness, family history, etc.) facilitates the communication, but knowing the generic expression for a special phrase is often necessary. For example, "short of breath walking up stairs" translates to "dyspnea on exertion." Because of the very large set of possible natural language phrases that might be encountered, such a translation is better made by the original observer than by the expert system.

An alternative scheme for structuring findings for use by an expert system would link "atoms" to "molecules" using a multiaxial dictionary such as is used by the Systematized Nomenclature of Medicine (SNOMED) system developed by the American College of Pathology.[75] Such a system allows more granularity to be expressed and does not require all usable phrases to be explicitly represented in the vocabulary. However, the user may enter terms not used in the knowledge base and be frustrated that the system does not know what to do with the information.

In the broad view, Iliad and other diagnostic medical expert systems must be linked to a patient database to make a significant difference in health care. A successful integration will greatly decrease the demand for data input from the user and will provide decision support using previously stored data (and decision support results) in combination with newly acquired data in a timely manner. Such a system must be able to differentiate outdated or inapproprate stored data from appropriate data, which will, in turn, require explicit handling of time. Such systems already exist (see Chapter 1) that can provide drug alerts, ICU monitoring, and various kinds of reminders, but none approaches the sophistication of Iliad, QMR, or DXplain.

A diagnostic expert system will only reach its full potential as a source of consultation in a patient care setting when it is able to communicate with other systems. In one study, an attempt was made to develop an interface between Iliad and HELP (an inpatient database that uses a structured vocabulary).[46] Several challenging problems were encountered even in this very modest experiment. Each data item in HELP is time stamped, and multiple examples of a given item such as hematocrit exist. Iliad, on the other hand, uses only the current value in most cases. To use data from HELP to drive the Iliad diagnostic system required not only the matching of terms in the two vocabularies but also developing algorithms for the common representation of the time course of events in the two systems.

Iliad represents knowledge specific to a given locale by adjusting the disease a priori probabilities. Further refinement of the model would also allow users to adjust the false positive statistics of some of the frames when large changes in a prioris are encountered. A worldwide web version of Iliad is currently in prototype and will allow for selection of appropriate probabilities for the environment of interest.

Diagnostic expert systems have a much wider range of uses than that of simply assigning diagnostic labels. Assistance in data collection, assessment of the quality of medical records, and extraction of relevant clinical data from natural language x-ray reports.[76] The Iliad expert system is being expanded into treatment, medical management, and risk management, as well as diagnosis. The KE tool included with this book can, in fact, be used to design expert systems that can support nonexperts in making any kind of decisions where available information is incomplete.

References

1. Reggia JA, Tuhrim S: An overview of methods for computer-assisted medical decision making. In: Reggia JA, Tuhrim F (eds) Computer-Assisted Medical Decision Making, Vol 1. New York: Springer-Verlag, 1985:3–37.
2. Miller PL: Artificial intelligence in medicine: an emerging discipline. In: Miller PL (ed) Selected Topics in Medical Artificial Intelligence. New York: Springer-Verlag, 1988:1–10.
3. Miller RA: Medical diagnostic decision support systems—past, present, and future. J Am Med Inf Assoc 1994;1:8–27.
4. Cahill BP, Holmen JR, Bartleson PL: Mayo Foundation electronic results inquiry, the HL7 connection. Proc Symp Comput Applications Med Care 1992;14:516–520.
5. Clayton PD, Pryor TA, Wigertz OB, Hripcsak G: Issues and structures for sharing medical knowledge among decision-making systems: the 1989 Arden Homestead Retreat. Proc Symp Comput Applications Med Care 1989;13:116–121.
6. Willems JL, Abreu-Lima C, Arnaud P, et al: The diagnostic performance of computer programs for the interpretation of electrocardiograms. N Engl J Med 1991;325:1767–1773.
7. Bartels PH, Thompson D, Weber JE: Expert systems in histopathology. IV. The management of uncertainty. Anal Quant Cytol Histol 1992;14:1–13.
8. Shortliffe EH, Buchanan BG, Feigenbaum EA: Knowledge engineering for medical decision-making: a review of computer-based clinical decision aids. Proc IEEE 1979;67:1207–1224.
9. Davis R, Buchanan B, Shoftliffe E: Production rules as a representation for a knowledge-based consultation program. In: Reggia JA, Tuhrim S (eds) Computer-Assisted Medical Decision Making, Vol 2. New York: Springer-Verlag, 1985:3–35.
10. McDonald CJ: Protocol-based computer reminders, the quality of care and the non-perfectability of man. N Engl J Med 1976;295:1351–1355.
11. Pryor TA, Gardner RM, Clayton PD, Warner HR: The HELP system. J Med Syst 1983;7:87–102.
12. Kuperman GJ, Gardner RM, Pryor TA: HELP: A Dynamic Hospital Information System. New York: Springer-Verlag, 1991.

13. Reggia JA: A production rule system for neurological localization. In: Reggia JA, Tuhrim S (eds) Computer-Assisted Medical Decision Making, Vol 2. New York: Springer-Verlag, 1985:49–62.
14. de Dombal FT, Leaper DJ, Staniland JR, McCann AP, Horrocks JC: Computer-aided diagnosis of acute abdominal pain. In: Reggia JA, Tuhrim S (eds) Computer-Assisted Medical Decision Making, Vol 1. New York: Springer-Verlag, 1985:159–169.
15. Warner HR, Toronot AF, Veasy LG: Experience with Bayes theorem for computer diagnosis of congenital heart disease. Ann NY Acad Sci 1964;115:2.
16. Zagoria R, Reggia J: Transferability of medical decision support based on Bayesian classification. Med Decision Making 1983;3:501–509.
17. Templeton A, Jensen C, Lehr J, Huff R: Solitary pulmonary lesions. Radiology 1967;89:605–613.
18. Overall JE, Williams CM: Conditional probability program for diagnosis of thyroid function. JAMA 1963;183:5.
19. Gorry GA, Barnett GO: Experience with a model of sequential diagnosis. In: Reggia JA, Tuhrim S (eds) Computer-Assisted Medical Decision Making, Vol 1. New York: Springer-Verlag, 1985:206–222.
20. Lichtenstein S: Conditional non-independence of data in a practical Bayesian decision task. Organ Behav Hum Perf 1972;8:2–25.
21. Ben-Bassat M, Carlson RW, Puri VK, Davenport MD, Schriver JA, Latif M, Smith R, Portigal LD, Lipnick EH, Weil MH: Pattern-based interactive diagnosis of multiple disorders: the MEDAS system. In: Reggia JA, Tuhrim S (eds) Computer-Assisted Medical Decision Making, Vol 1. New York: Springer-Verlag, 1985:223–250.
22. Li Y-C, Haug PJ: Evaluating the quality of a probabilistic diagnostic system using different inferencing strategies. Proc Symp Comput Applications Med Care 1993;17:471–477.
23. Shwe M, Middleton B, Heckerman D, Henrion M, Horvitz E, Lehmann H, Cooper G: A probabilistic reformulation of the Quick Medical Reference system. Proc Symp Comput Applications Med Care 1990;14:790–794.
24. Rutledge GW, Andersen SK, Polaschek JX, Fagan LM: A belief network model for interpretation of ICU data. Proc Symp Comput Applications Med Care 1990;14:785–788.
25. Pearl J: Bayesian belief networks, also referred to as probabilistic causal networks or Bayesian networks. Evidential reasoning using stochastic stimulation of causal models. Artif Intell 1987;32:245–252.
26. Kulikowski CA: Problems in the design of knowledge bases for medical consultation. In: Reggia JA, Tuhrim S (eds) Computer-Assisted Medical Decision Making, Vol 2. New York: Springer-Verlag, 1985:38–48.
27. Miller RA, People HE Jr, Myers JD: INTERNIST-1, an expierimental computer-based diagnostic consultant for general internal medicine. In: Reggia JA, Tuhrim S (eds) Computer-Assisted Medical Decision Making, Vol 2. New York: Spring-Verlag, 1985:139–158.
28. Miller RA, Masarie FE, Myers JD: Quick Medical Reference (QMR) for diagnostic assistance. MD Comput 1986;3:34–48.
29. Miller RA, Masarie FE: Quick Medical Reference (QMR): an evolving, microcomputer-based diagnostic decision-support program for general internal medicine. Proc Symp Comput Applications Med Care 1989;13:947–951.

30. Feldman MJ, Barnett GO: An approach to evaluating the accuracy of DXplain. Proc Symp Comput Applications Med Care 1990;14:38–43.
31. Packer MS, Hoffer EP, Barnett GO, Famiglietti KT, Kim RJ, McLatchey JP, Elkin PL, Cimino C, Studney DR: Evolution of DXplain: a decision support system. Proc Symp Comput Applications Med Care 1989;13:949–951.
32. Warner HR, Haug PJ, Bouhaddou O, Lincoln MJ, Warner HR Jr, Sorenson DK, Williamson JW, Fan C: ILIAD as an expert consultant to teach differential diagnosis. Proc Symp Comput Applications Med Care 1988;12:371–376.
33. Sorenson DK, Bouhaddou O, Wange W, Canfield G, Fu L, Warner HR: Generation and maintenance of Iliad medical knowledge in a HyperCard environment. Proc Symp Comput Applications Med Care 1989;12:366–370.
34. Yu H, Haug PJ, Lincoln MJ, Turner C, Warner HR: Clustered knowledge representation: increasing the reliability of computerized expert systems. Proc Symp Comput Applications Med Care 1988;12:126–130.
35. Sorenson DK, Cundick RM, Fan C, Warner HR: Passing partial information among Bayesean and Boolean frames. Proc Symp Comput Applications Med Care 1989;13:50–56.
36. Bouhaddou O, Warner HR, Yu H, Lincoln MJ: The knowledge capabilites of the vocabulary component of a medical expert system. Proc Symp Comput Applications Med Care 1990;14:655–659.
37. Fu LS, Bouhaddou O, Huff SM, Sorenson DK, Warner HR: Toward A public domain UMLS patient database. Proc Symp Comput Applications Med Care 1990;14:170–174.
38. First MB, Williams JBW, Spitzer RL: DTREE: microcomputer-assisted traching of psychiatric diagnosis using a decision tree model. Proc Symp Comput Applications Med Care 1988;12:377–381.
39. Warner HR: Medical informatics: a real discipline? J Am Med Inf Assoc 1995;2:207–214.
40. Weinstein MC, Fineberg HV: Clinical Decision Analysis. Philadelphia: Saunders, 1980.
41. Lehmann HP, Shortliffe EH: THOMAS: building Bayesian statistical expert systems to aid in clinical decision making. Proc Symp Comput Applications Med Care 1990;14:58–64.
42. Lobodzinski SM, Laks MM: Present and future concepts in computerized electrocardiography. Arrhythmia Clin 1987;3/3:31–48.
43. Fries JF, McShane DJ: ARAMIS (the American rheumatism association medical information system). West J Med 1986;145:798–804.
44. McDonald CJ, Tierney WM, Overhage JM, Martin DK, Wilson GA: The Regenstrief medical record system: 20 years of experience in hospitals, clinics, and neighborhood health centers. MD Comput 1992;9:206–217.
45. Barnett GO: The application of computer-based medical-record systems in ambulatory practice. N Engl J Med 1984;310:1643–1650.
46. Wong ET, Pryor TA, Huff SM, Haug PJ, Warner HR: Interfacing a stand-alone diagnostic expert system with a hospital information system. Comput Biomed Res 1994;27:116–129.
47. Lincoln MJ, Turner CW, Haug PJ, Warner HR, Williamson JW, Bouhaddou O, Jessen SG, Sorenson D, Cundick RC, Grant M: Ilaid training enhances medical students' diagnostic skills. J Med Syst 1991;14:93–110.

48. Warner HR: Computer-Assisted Medical Decision Making. New York: Academic Press, 1979.
49. Rocha RA, Huff SM, Haug PJ, Warner HR: Designing a controlled medical vocabulary server: the VOSER project. Comput Biomed Res 1994;27:472–507.
50. Kassirer JP, Kopelman RI: Diagnosis and decisions by algorithms. Hosp Pract (Off Ed) 1990;25:23–24, 27, 31.
51. Ben Said M, Dougherty N, Anderson C, Altman SJ, Bouhaddou O, Warner HR: KESS: knowledge engineering support system. Symp Comput Applications Med Care 1987;11:56–59.
52. Giuse DA, Giuse NB, Miller RA: KB editing with QMR-KAT. Symp Comput Applications Med Care 1993;17:935.
53. Huff SM, Craig RB, Gould BL, Castagno DL, Smilan RE: Medical data dictionary for decision support applications. Proc Annu Symp Comput Applications Med Care 1987;11:310–317.
54. Rennels GD, Shortliffe EH, Miller PL: Choice and explanation in medical management: a multiattribute model of artificial intelligence approaches. Med Decision Making 1987;7:22–31.
55. Guo D, Lincoln MJ, Haug PJ, Turner CW, Warner HR: Exploring a new best information algorithm for Iliad. Proc Symp Comput Applications Med Care 1992;16:624–628.
56. Turner CW, Williamson J, Lincoln MJ, Haug PJ, Buchanan J, Anderson C, Grant M, Cundick R, Warner HR: The effects of Iliad on medical student problem solving. Proc Symp Comput Applications Med Care 1990;14:478–482.
57. Cundick R, Turner CW, Lincoln MJ, Buchanan JP, Anderson C, Warner HR, Bouhaddou O: Iliad as a patient case stimulator to teach medical problem solving. Proc Symp Comput Applications Med Care 1989;13:902–906.
58. Turner CW, Lincoln MJ, Haug P, Williamson JW, Jessen S, Cundick K, Warner HR: Iliad training effects: a cognitive model and empirical findings. Proc Symp Comput Applications Med Care 1992;16:68–72.
59. Huff SM, Rocha RA, Bray BE, Warner HR, Haug PJ: An event model of medical information representation. J Am Inf Assoc 1995;2:116–134.
60. Cimino JJ, Johnson SB, Peng P, Aguirre A: From ICD9-CM to MeSH using the UMLS. Symp Comput Applications Med Care 1993;17:730–734.
61. Physicians' Current Procedure Terminology, 1995. Chicago: American Medical Association, 1995.
62. Stensaas SS, Bouhaddou O, Hardy L, Sorenson DK, Dougherty NE, Altman SJ: The educational potential of linking a videodisc and an expert system. Proc Symp Comput Applications Med Care 1989;13:864–868.
63. Pryor TA: Electrocardiographic interpretation by computer. Comput Biomed Res 1969;2:537–548.
64. Hripcsak G, Clayton PD, Pryor TA, Haug P, Wigertz OB, Van der lei J: The Arden syntax for medical logic modules. Proc Annu Symp Comput Applications Med Care 1990;14:200–204.
65. Kratzer MA, Ivandic B, Fateh-Moghadam A: Neuronal network analysis of serum electrophoresis. J Clin Pathol 1992;45:612–615.
66. Bouhaddou O, Frucci L, Cofrin K, Larsen D, Warner HR Jr, Huber P, Sorenson DK, Turner C, Warner HR: Implementation of practice guidelines in a clinical setting using a computerized knowledge base (Iliad). Proc Symp Comput Applications Med Care 1993;17:258–262.

67. Lau LM, Warner HR: Performance of a diagnostic system (Iliad) as a tool for quality assurance. Comput Biomed Res 1992;25:314–323.
68. Fisher RC. Patient education and compliance: a pharmacist's perspective. Patient Educ Counsel 1992;19,3:261–271.
69. Forman L: Medication: reasons and interventions for noncompliance. J Psychosoc Nurs Health Serv 1993;31(10):23–25.
70. Kahn G: Computer-based patient education: a progress report. MD Comput 1993;10(2):93–99.
71. America's compliance problem. National Council on Patient Information and Education, Washington, DC.
72. Carrell S: Overview and Summary of the First National Conference on Consumer Health Informatics, Stevens Point, WI, July 17–18, 1993.
73. Bouhaddou O, Lepage E, Huber P: Challenges in disseminating a probability-based expert system: the French and German versions of Iliad®. Proceedings of MedInfo'92, Geneva, Switzerland, 1992.
74. Kuperman GJ, James BC, Jacobsen JT, Gardner RM: Continuous quality improvement applied to medical care: experience at LDS Hospital. Med Decision Making 1991;11:S60–S65.
75. Rothwell DJ, Cote RA: Optimizing the structure of a standardized vocabulary: the SNOMED model. Proc Symp Comput Applications Med Care 1990;14:181–184.
76. Haug PJ: Uses of diagnostic expert systems in clinical care. Proc Symp Comput Applications Med Care 1993;17:379–383.

Appendix 1
Example Hierarchies of Final Diagnoses of Top-Level Diseases in Various Medical Specialties

Note that in this list, "+" indicates a heading, not a top-level disease.

CARDIOVASCULAR DISORDERS

+Arrhythmias
  AV (atrioventricular) block (2nd or 3rd degree)
  Digitalis toxicity
  +Supraventricular arrhythmias
    Atrial fibrillation/flutter
    Atrial septal defect
    Lown–Ganong–Levine syndrome
    Multifocal atrial tachycardia (MAT)
    Paroxysmal supraventricular tachycardia (PSVT)
    Sick sinus syndrome
    Wolff–Parkinson–White syndrome
  +Ventricular arrhythmias
    Long Q-T syndrome
    Ventricular tachycardia
+Cardiac trauma
  Myocardial contusion
+Cardiomyopathy
  Fibromuscular dysplasia
  Heart failure
    Right-sided heart failure
    Left-sided heart failure
    Cardiogenic shock
  +Dilated cardiomyopathy
    Alcoholic cardiomyopathy
    Beriberi heart disease
    Chagas' disease

    Ischemic cardiomyopathy
    Peripartum cardiomyopathy
    Idiopathic cardiomyopathy
  Hypertrophic cardiomyopathy
  Myocarditis
  Restrictive cardiomyopathy
    Carcinoid heart disease
    Loeffler's endocarditis
    Myocardial fibrosis; radiation induced
  Myxedema heart disease
  Thyrotoxic heart disease
+Congenital
  Atrial septal defect
  Coarctation of the aorta
  Eisenmenger's syndrome
  Patent ductus arteriosus
  Supravalvular aortic stenosis
  Tetralogy of Fallot
  Tricuspid atresia
  VSD (ventricular septal defect)
+Coronary artery disease
  Acute MI (myocardial infarction)
  +Angina
    Stable angina
    Unstable angina
  Coronary artery spasm
  Left ventricular aneurysm
+Hypertension
  Drug-induced hypertension
  Essential hypertension
  Hypertensive heart disease
  Malignant hypertension
  Renovascular hypertension
+Pericardial disorders
  Malignant pericardial effusion
  Pericarditis; bacterial
  Pericarditis; constrictive
  Pericarditis; postmyocardial infarction (Dressler's)
  Pericarditis; tuberculous
  Pneumopericardium
  Postcardiotomy syndrome
  Cardiac tamponade
+Tumors
  +Myxoma
    Atrial myxoma; left

Atrial myxoma; right
+Valvular disorders
  Mitral stenosis
  Aortic insufficiency
  +Mitral regurgitation
    Mitral regurgitation; chronic
    Mitral regurgitation; acute
  Aortic stenosis
  Atrial septal defect
  Mitral valve prolapse
  Pulmonic stenosis
  Pulmonic insufficiency
  Ruptured abdominal aortic aneurysm
  Status post heart valve replacement
  Tricuspid regurgitation
  Tricuspid stenosis
  Tricuspid prolapse

+Arterial diseases
  +Obliterative arterial disease
    Arteriosclerosis obliterans (peripheral vascular disease)
    Leriche syndrome (thrombosis of aorta before the bifurcation)
    Thromboangiitis obliterans (Buerger's disease)
  +Arterial aneurysmal disease
    +Aortic aneurysms
      Ruptured abdominal aortic aneurysm
      Thoracic aortic aneurysm
    Aortic dissection
  +Arterial thromboembolic disease
    Blue toes syndrome
    Peripheral arterial embolism
  +Arterial injury in general
    Arteriovenous (AV) fistula
    Blunt and penetrating trauma
    Chemical injury
    False aneurysm
    Thermal injury
  +Vasospastic arterial disease
  +Inflammatory and collagen vascular disease
  +Arterial compression syndromes
  +Organ arterial insufficiencies

+Venous diseases
  +Thrombophlebitis (venous thrombosis)

Deep venous thrombophlebitis of extremity
Superficial thrombophlebitis of extremity
Thrombophlebitis of communicating veins of extremity
Pelvic vein thrombophlebitis
Venous thrombosis in the upper extremities
    Paget–von Schroetter disease
Venous thromboembolism
Chronic venous insufficiency
    Venous incompetence
    +Varicose veins
        Varicose vein(s); primary
        Varicose vein(s); secondary
    Postphlebitic syndrome
+Trauma (blunt or penetrating) venous problems
+Caval obstruction syndromes
+Special organ venous problems
    Mesenteric venous thrombosis
Klippel–Trenaunay syndrome

+Lymphatic diseases
    +Lymphedema
        Lymphedema; primary
        Lymphedema; secondary
    Lymphangitis
    Lymphadenitis
    Lymphatic fistula
    +Lymphatic vessel tumors; benign
        Lymphangioma
        Cystic hygroma

+General vascular diseases
    +Malignant vascular tumors
        Angiosarcoma (lymphangiosarcoma or hemangiosarcoma)
    Vascular gangrene

DERMATOLOGIC DISORDERS

+Alopecia
    +Scarring
        Discoid lupus erythematosus
        Kerion
        Folliculitis decalvans
        Lichen planopilaris
        Pseudopalade of Brocq

+Nonscarring
  Alopecia areata
  Alopecia trichotillomania
  Androgenetic alopecia
  +Hair shaft abnormalities
  Metabolic alopecia
  Telogen effluvium
  Traction alopecia
+Bites and stings; insect
  Bee or wasp sting
  Insect bite
  Spider bite
+Bites and stings; noninsect
  Dog bites
  Human bite
  Snake bite
+Developmental skin disorders
  +Cutaneous vascular malformation
    Cavernous/capillary hemangioma
    Port wine stain
+Drug-induced skin disease
  Drug-induced erythema multiforme
    Toxic epidermal necrolysis (TEN)
  Drug-induced hyperpigmentation
  Drug-induced photosensitivity
  Drug-induced morbilliform rash
  Fixed drug reaction
+Eczematous diseases
  Atopic dermatitis
  Contact dermatitis
  Dyshidrotic eczema
  Lichen simplex chronicus
  Nummular eczema
  Seborrheic dermatitis
  Stasis dermatitis
  Xerosis
+Fungal diseases
  Cutaneous candidiasis
  +Dermatophytes
    Kerion
    Tinea cruris
    Tinea corporis
    Tinea capitis
    Tinea pedis
    Tinea versicolor

+Deep fungal
  Skin lesion of blastomycosis
  Skin lesion of coccidiodomycosis
  Skin lesion of histoplasmosis
+Infectious skin diseases
  Carbunculosis or furunculosis
  Cellulitis
  Chancroid
  Cutaneous anthrax
  Erysipelas
  Erythrasma
  Folliculitis
  Genital herpes simplex
  Herpes zoster
  Hot tub folliculitis
  Impetigo
  Molluscum contagiosum
  Orf
  Swimming pool granuloma (*Mycobacterium marinum*)
  Wart
    Condyloma (genital wart)
+Infestations
  +Lice (crabs)
    Body lice (pediculosis corporis)
    Head lice (pediculosis capitis)
    Pubic lice (pediculosis pubis)
  Scabies
  Swimmers' itch
+Keratinization disorders
  Benign familial pemphigus
  Darier's disease (keratosis follicularis)
  Grover's disease (transient acantholytic dermatosis)
  +Ichthyosis
    Bullous ichthyosiform erythroderma (epidermolytic
            hyperkeratosis)
    Lamellar ichthyosis
    X-linked ichthyosis
    Ichthyosis vulgaris
  Palmar/plantar keratoderma
+Neurocutaneous disorders
  Hereditary hemorrhagic telangiectasia (Osler–Weber–Rendu)
  Neurofibromatosis I
  Neurofibromatosis II
  Tuberous sclerosis
+Oral skin disorders

Canker sore (aphthous stomatitis)
+Papulosquamous diseases
  Pityriasis rosea
  Lichen planus
  Psoriasis (plaque psoriasis)
      Psoriasis; guttate
  Syphilis; secondary
  Tinea corporis
+Paronychia
  Bacterial paronychia
  Candida paronychia
+Photodermatitis
  Allergic contact photosensitivity
  Drug-induced photosensitivity
  Polymorphous light eruption
  Solar urticaria
  Sunburn
+Pigmentation disorders
  Melasma
  Postinflammatory hyperpigmentation
  Postinflammatory hypopigmentation
  Vitiligo
+Pustular diseases
  Acne
  Rosacea
+Tumors
  +Benign skin tumors
    Cherry angioma
    Cutaneous cyst
    Dermatofibroma
    Keloid
    Lipoma
    Nevi (mole)
        Congenital nevi [bathing suit nevi, giant-hairy nevi]
    Sebaceous gland hyperplasia
    Seborrheic keratosis
    Skin tag (acrochordon)
    Solitary neurofibroma
    Xanthoma
  +Malignant skin tumors
    Actinic keratosis
    Basal cell carcinoma
        Basal cell carcinoma; morpheaform
    Squamous cell carcinoma
    Melanoma

      Acral lentiginous melanoma
      Lentigo maligna melanoma
      Nodular melanoma
      Superficial spreading melanoma
    Keratoacanthoma
  +Cutaneous manifestations of malignancy
    Cutaneous non-T-cell lymphoma
    Leukemia cutis
    Metastatic cutaneous malignancy
    Mycosis fungoides (cutaneous T-cell lymphoma)
+Vascular reactions
  Angioedema
  Dermatomyositis
  Discoid lupus erythematosus
  Erythema multiforme
  Subacute cutaneous lupus erythematosus
  Systemic sclerosis (scleroderma)
  Urticaria
  +Vasculitis-related skin diseases
    Allergic vasculitis
    Necrotizing vasculitis
  Viral exanthem
+Vesiculobullous diseases
  Bullous pemphigoid
  +Epidermolysis bullosa (EB)
    EB dystrophic
    EB simplex
    EB junctional
  Pemphigus vulgaris
  Porphyria cutanea tarda
+Miscellaneous skin diseases
  Acanthosis nigricans
  Granuloma annulare
  +Panniculitis
    Cutaneous signs of acute pancreatitis
    Erythema nodosum
  Sweet's syndrome

ENDOCRINE AND METABOLIC DISORDERS

+Pituitary
  Acromegaly
  Diabetes insipidus; central
  Pituitary Cushing's (Cushing's disease)
    Nelson's syndrome

Pituitary tumor
Hypopituitarism
   Pituitary adrenal insufficiency
   Hypogonadotrophic hypogonadism (Kallman's syndrome)
+Prolactinoma
   Prolactinoma—females
   Prolactinoma—males
Empty sella syndrome
+Thyroid
  +Thyroid tumor
   Anaplastic carcinoma of the thyroid
   Colloid nodular goiter
   Follicular tumor of the thyroid (adenoma or carcinoma)
   Papillary carcinoma of the thyroid
   Medullary carcinoma of thyroid
   Thyroid lymphoma
  Hyperthyroidism
   Graves' disease
   Painless (silent) thyroiditis
   Subacute thyroiditis
   Thyrotoxic periodic paralysis
   Thyrotoxic storm
   Toxic nodular goiter
  Hypothyroidism
   Congenital hypothyroidism
   Chronic thyroiditis (Hashimoto's disease)
   Hypothyroidism; primary
   Hypothyroidism; secondary
   Drug-induced hypothyroidism
   Myxedema coma
  Euthyroid sick syndrome
  Hyperthyroxinemia without hyperthyroidism
  Thyroid hemorrhage
+Parathyroid
  Hypoparathyroidism
  +Hyperparathyroidism
   Primary hyperparathyroidism
   Severe secondary hyperparathyroidism
   Mild secondary hyperparathyroidism
   Hypercalcemia of malignancy
  Pseudohypoparathyroidism
+Adrenal
  +Adrenal insufficiency
   Acute adrenal crisis
   Addison's disease

   Adrenal apoplexy
   Exogenous adrenal insufficiency
Adrenoleukodystrophy
CAH (congenital adrenal hyperplasia) (female; classical)
CAH (female; nonclassical)
+Cushing's syndrome
   Cushing's syndrome caused by adrenal tumor
   Ectopic Cushing's syndrome
   Cushing's syndrome; exogenous
Nonfunctional adrenal carcinoma or adenoma
Nonfunctional benign adrenal mass
Pheochromocytoma
Primary hyperaldosteronism
Salt-losing congenital adrenal hyperplasia
Testosterone-producing adrenal adenoma
+Pancreas
   +Diabetes
      NIDDM (non-insulin-dependent diabetes mellitus)
      IDDM (insulin-dependent diabetes mellitus)
      Diabetic hyperglycemic hyperosmolar coma
      Diabetic ketoacidosis
      Diabetic neuropathy
      Diabetic nephropathy
   Islet of Langerhans tumor
      Gastrinoma (Zollinger–Ellison syndrome)
      Glucagonoma
      Insulinoma
      VIPoma
+Gonadal; female
   Autoimmune ovarian failure
   Polycystic ovary syndrome
   Turner's syndrome
+Gonadal; male
   Klinefelter's syndrome
   Testicular failure
   +Testicular tumors
      Leydig cell tumor
      Seminoma
      Nonseminoma testicular tumor
+Hyperlipoproteinemias
   Chylomicronemia syndrome
   Familial combined hyperlipidemia
   Familial dysbetalipoproteinemia
   Familial hypercholesterolemia
   Familial hypertriglyceridemia

Familial lipoprotein lipase deficiency
Hyperlipidemia; acquired
Hypertriglyceridemia; sporadic
Polygenic hypercholesterolemia
+Multiple endocrine abnormalities
  +Multiple endocrine neoplasias (MEN)
    MEN I
    MEN II
+Metabolic disorders
  Alcoholic ketoacidosis
  Anorexia nervosa
  Bulimia
  Carcinoid syndrome
  Cystinosis
  Cystinuria
  Ethylene glycol intoxication
  Fanconi's syndrome; acquired
  Fanconi's syndrome; familial
  Familial Mediterranean fever
  Fructose intolerance
  Fructose-1,6-diphosphatase deficiency
  Galactosemia (due to transferase deficiency)
  Galactosemia (due to kinase deficiency)
  Hartnup's disease
  Hemochromatosis
  Hereditary amyloidosis
  Hereditary urea cycle abnormality
  +Homocystinuria
    Cystathionine beta-synthetase deficiency
  Hyperornithinemia
  Hypoglycemia
  Lactic acidosis
  Malnutrition
  Maple syrup urine disease
  Methanol intoxication
  Methylmalonic acidemia
  Oncogenic osteomalacia
  Osteomalacia
  Osteoporosis (symptomatic)
  Oxalosis
  Propionic acidemia
  +Tyrosinemia
    Hereditary tyrosinemia I
  Tyrosinosis
+Nutritional deficiencies and toxicities

    Diet-associated ketoacidosis
    Folate deficiency
    Osteomalacia
    Pellagra (niacin deficiency)
    Pernicious anemia
    Pyridoxine (vitamin B_6) deficiency
    Rickets
    Scurvy
    Thiamine deficiency (beriberi)
    Vitamin A deficiency
    Vitamin A toxicity
    Vitamin B_2 deficiency
    Vitamin D toxicity
    Vitamin K deficiency
+Electrolyte disorders
    Bartter's syndrome
    Dilutional hyponatremia
    Ectopic SIADH (syndrome of inappropriate antidiuretic
                hormone)
    Hyperkalemic periodic paralysis (adynamia)
    Hypomagnesemia
    Hypophosphatemia
    Hyporenenemic hypoaldosteronism
    Milk alkali syndrome
    Periodic paralysis with hypokalemia
    Thyrotoxic periodic paralysis
+Miscellaneous
    Adrenogenital syndrome
    Albinism
    Carcinoid syndrome
    Drug-induced hypoglycemia
    Facticious hypoglycemia
    Fabry's disease
    +Glycogen storage diseases
       McArdle's syndrome (glycogen storage disease type V)
       Von Gierke's disease
    Lead poisoning
    Morbid obesity
    Congenital generalized lipodystrophy
    Acquired generalized lipodystrophy
    Partial lipodystrophy

GASTROINTESTINAL DISORDERS (GI)

+Esophageal disorders
    Bleeding esophageal varices

Esophageal stricture (benign)
+Esophageal motility disorders
  Esophageal spasm
  Achalasia
Lower esophageal ring (Schatzki's)
Esophageal cancer
Esophageal perforation
Gastroesophageal reflux disease
+Gastroduodenal disorders
  +Peptic ulcer disease
    Gastric ulcer; benign
    Duodenal ulcer
      Gastric outlet obstruction
  +Gastritis
    Gastritis; acute
    Stress gastritis
    Helicobacter pylori gastritis (chronic gastritis)
    Chronic autoimmune gastritis (atrophic gastritis)
    Giant hypertrophic gastritis (Menetrier's disease)
  Gastric cancer
  Mallory–Weiss tear
  Gastroparesis
+Intestinal disorders
  Acute appendicitis
  Acute colonic pseudo-obstruction (Ogilivie's syndrome)
  Adenocarcinoma of the small bowel
  Adenomatous small bowel polyp
  Angiodysplasia of the GI tract
  Chronic intestinal pseudoobstruction
  Colon cancer
  Colorectal polyps ≥1 cm
  +Diarrhea
    +Osmotic diarrhea
      +Malabsorption
        +Luminal digestive defects
          Pancreatic malabsorption
        +Mucosal malabsorption
          Celiac disease (sprue)
          Tropical sprue
          Lactase deficiency
          Short bowel syndrome
        +Micellar defect
          Intestinal bacterial overgrowth (blind loop syndrome)
          Bile salt malabsorption
        +Intestinal delivery defect
          +Intestinal lymphatic obstruction

           Whipple's disease
           Intestinal lymphangiectasia
        Iatrogenic diarrhea
        Protein-losing gastroenteropathy
        +Secretory diarrhea
          Cholera
          Staphylococcus aureus food poisoning
        +Humoral (endocrine tumors)
          Vipoma
          Gastrinoma (Zollinger–Ellison syndrome)
        +Luminal stimuli
          Bile salt malabsorption
      +Motility disorders
        Irritable bowel syndrome (functional bowel)
        Dumping syndrome
      +Multifactorial
        +Inflammatory diarrhea
          +Inflammatory bowel disease
            Ulcerative colitis
              Toxic megacolon
            Crohn's disease; regional enteritis
            +Infectious inflammatory diarrhea
              Bacterial gastroenteritis
                Salmonella enteritis
                Shigella enteritis
                E. coli enteritis
                Campylobacter enteritis
                Pseudomembranous colitis
            Viral gastroenteritis
          +Parasitic
            Giardiasis
          Amebiasis
      Radiation enteritis
      Ischemic colitis
    Diverticular colonic bleed
    Diverticulitis
    Diverticulosis
    Fecal impaction
    Gastrointestinal perforation
    Hemorrhoids
    Intestinal leiomyoma
    Intestinal obstruction
    Intraabdominal abscess
    Meckel's diverticulum
    Pneumatosis cystoides intestinalis

Polyposis syndrome; familial
+Hepatic disorders
+Hepatocellular jaundice
+Acute viral hepatitis
Hepatitis A
Hepatitis B
Hepatitis C
Delta agent (hepatitis D)
+Chronic hepatitis
Chronic active hepatitis
Chronic persistent hepatitis
Autoimmune hepatitis
+Toxic hepatocellular jaundice
Alcoholic liver disease (hepatitis/cirrhosis)
Drug-induced hepatitis
Nonalcoholic steatohepatitis
Ischemic hepatocellular jaundice
Intrahepatic cholestasis of pregnancy
Fatty liver of pregnancy
+Cirrhosis
Alcoholic liver disease (hepatitis/cirrhosis)
Postnecrotic cirrhosis
Liver failure
Bleeding esophageal varices
Hepatic encephalopathy
+Masses
Hepatic focal nodular hyperplasia
Hepatic hemangioma
Hepatocellular adenoma
Hepatocellular carcinoma
Liver metastases
+Liver abscess
Amebic liver abscess
Pyogenic liver abscess
+Intrahepatic
Drug-induced cholestasis
Primary biliary cirrhosis
Hepatic vein obstruction (Budd–Chiari)
Peliosis hepatis
Polycystic liver disease
+Unconjugated hyperbilirubinemia
Gilbert's syndrome
Crigler–Najjar disease; type I
Crigler–Najjar disease; type II
+Conjugated hyperbilirubinemia

Dubin–Johnson syndrome
+Biliary disorders
  +Cholestatic jaundice
    +Biliary obstruction
      +Stones
        Acute cholangitis
        Acute cholecystitis
        Choledocholithiasis
        Cholelithiasis
        Chronic cholecystitis
      +Tumors
        Cholangiocarcinoma
      Biliary stricture
      Sphincter of Oddi dysfunction
  +Strictures
    Sclerosing cholangitis
+Pancreatic disorders
  Acute pancreatitis
  Chronic pancreatitis
    Pancreatic pseudocyst
    Pancreatic malabsorption
  Pancreatic abscess
  Pancreatic carcinoma

OBSTETRICAL AND GYNECOLOGICAL DISORDERS (OB/GYN)

+Obstetrics
  Abortion; threatened
    +Abortion; spontaneous
      Abortion; inevitable
      Abortion; incomplete
      Abortion; complete
      Abortion; infected
    Abortion; missed
  +Complicated pregnancy
    Pregnancy with rubella
    Pregnancy with positive herpes
    Pregnancy with positive hepatitis
    Pregnancy with positive VDRL and FTA
    Pregnancy with positive HIV (human immunodeficiency virus)
    Pregnancy with Rh– mother and Rh+ father
  Dead fetus syndrome
  Ectopic pregnancy
  First-trimester pregnancy
  Gestational diabetes

Multiple gestation
Possible fetal alcohol syndrome
Postpartum hemorrhage
+Pregnancy-induced hypertension
  Preeclampsia
  Eclampsia
  HELLP syndrome
Third-trimester bleeding
  Placenta abruptio
    Placenta abruptio with fetal distress
  Placenta previa
+Gynecology
  +Abnormal uterine bleeding
    Anovulatory (dysfunctional uterine) bleeding
    +Peri- or postmenopausal bleeding
      Atrophic vaginitis
      Iatrogenic postmenopausal bleeding
  +Gynecological cancers
    Cancer of the vulva
    Cervical cancer
    Endometrial cancer
    Ovarian cancer
    +Trophoblastic disease
      Hydatidiform mole
      Choriocarcinoma
    +Uterine cancer
      Leiomyosarcoma
    Vaginal cancer
  +Gynecological infections
    Pelvic inflammatory disease (PID)
    Trichomoniasis
    Postpartum endometritis
    Vaginal yeast infection
    Vulvovaginitis
  +General gynecological problems
    Bartholin's abscess or cyst
    Cervical dysplasia
    Developmental disorders of the cervix, uterus, and fallopian
          tubes
    Developmental disorders of the vagina and vulva
    Endometriosis
    Fibroid (uterine leiomyoma)
    Imperforate hymen
    Premenstrual syndrome
    Ruptured ovarian cyst

Stress incontinence
Uterine prolapse
Urethral prolapse
+Breast problems
Breast cancer
+Benign breast disease
Fibrocystic breast disease
Mastitis
+Breast prosthesis complications
Breast abscess

HEMATOLOGICAL DISORDERS

+Anemia
Anemia of chronic disease
Anemia of endocrine disease
+Aplastic anemia
Idiopathic aplastic anemia
Secondary aplastic anemia
Hemolytic anemia
Hereditary spherocytosis
Sickle cell anemia
Clinical hemoglobin C
Hemolytic anemia due to G6PD (glucose-6-phosphate
dehydrogenase) deficiency
Immune hemolytic anemia
Idiopathic autoimmune hemolytic anemia
Secondary immune hemolytic anemia
Paroxysmal cold hemoglobinuria (PCH)
Nonimmune hemolytic anemia caused by chemical or physical
agents
Drug-induced immune hemolytic anemia
Paroxysmal nocturnal hemoglobinuria (PNH)
Hereditary elliptocytosis
Hereditary ovalocytosis
+Microcytic anemia
Iron deficiency anemia
Clinical thalassemia (major and minor)
Thalassemia minor (alpha)
Thalassemia minor (beta)
+Megaloblastic anemia
Anemia of B_{12} deficiency
Pernicious anemia
Anemia of folate deficiency
+Hemologinopathies

   Sickle cell anemia
   Clinical hemoglobin C
   Rare hemoglobinopathies
   Polycythemia due to high oxygen affinity Hgb (Hb)
+Leukemias
 Acute lymphocytic leukemia
 Acute nonlymphocytic leukemia
 Chronic lymphocytic leukemia (CLL)
 Chronic myelocytic leukemia (CML)
  CML in myeloblastic/lymphoblastic crisis
 Chronic myelomonocytic leukemia (CMML)
 Hairy cell leukemia
+Lymphomas
 Hodgkin's lymphoma
 Non-Hodgkin's lymphoma
+Gammopathies (hyperviscosity syndromes)
 Multiple myeloma
 Macroglobulinemia of Waldenstrom
 Light chain disease
 +Amyloid diseases
  +Systemic amyloid
   Primary amyloid
   Secondary systemic amyloid
  Cardiac amyloid
  Amyloid following chronic hemodialysis
 Monoclonal gammopathy of unknown significance
 Cold hyperviscosity syndrome
  Primary cryoglobulinemia
  Secondary cryoglobulinemia
 +Hyperviscosity syndrome (non-thermal-related)
  Primary hyperviscosity syndrome
  Secondary hyperviscosity syndrome
Myelodysplastic syndrome (refractory anemia)
 RAEB (refractory anemia with excess blasts)
 RAEB-T (refractory anemia excess blasts in transition)
 RARS (refractory anemia with ringed sideroblasts)
 Secondary myelodysplasia (acute myelodysplasia)
 Chronic myelomonocytic leukemia (CMML)
Myelophthisic process
 Primary myelofibrosis (agnogenic myeloid metaplasia)
 Myelophthisic process due to cancer
 Myelophthisic process due to granuloma
+Polycythemia
 Polycythemia vera
 Polycythemia (erythrocytosis) due to hypoxemia

    Polycythemia due to erythropoietin excess without hypoxemia
    Polycythemia due to high oxygen affinity Hb
    Relative ("spurious"; "Gaisbock's") polycythemia
+Bleeding disorders
  Primary fibrinolysis
  +Coagulopathies
    +Hemophilia
      Factor I (fibrinogen) deficiency
      Factor II (prothrombin) deficiency
      Factor V deficiency
      Factor VII deficiency
      Hemophilia A (factor VIII deficiency)
      Hemophilia B (factor IX deficiency)
      Factor X deficiency
      Factor XI deficiency
      Factor XII (Hageman factor) deficiency
      Factor XIII deficiency
    +Von Willebrand's disease
      Type I von Willebrand's disease
      Type II von Willebrand's disease
    +Anticoagulant defects
      Congenital protein C or S deficiency
      Congenital antithrombin III deficiency
      Acquired antithrombin III deficiency
      Lupus anticoagulant
    DIC (disseminated intravascular coagulation) (consumption
        coagulopathy)
    Hemolytic uremic syndrome
    Drug-induced vitamin K deficiency
  +Platelet disorders
    Congenital platelet function defect
    Acquired platelet function defect
    +Thrombocythemia
      Primary thrombocythemia
    +Thrombocytopenia
      Thrombotic thrombocytopenic purpura (TTP)
      Idiopathic thrombocytopenic purpura (ITP)
      +Drug-induced (secondary)
        Drug-induced immune thrombocytopenia
        Drug-induced nonimmune thrombocytopenia
+Infectious hematological diseases
  Infectious mononucleosis (CMV)
  Infectious mononucleosis (EB)
+Miscellaneous
  Cyclic neutropenia

Gaucher's disease
Methemoglobinemia; hereditary
Methemoglobinemia; acquired

INFECTIOUS DISEASES

+Intraabdominal infections
  Acute appendicitis
  +Peritonitis
    Peritonitis; spontaneous
    Peritonitis; secondary
    Peritonitis; dialysis-associated
+Intravascular infections
  Culture-negative endocarditis
  Infective endocarditis
  Sepsis
  Septic shock
  Septic thrombophlebitis
+Neurological infections
  Botulism
  Diphtheria
  +CNS (central nervous system) infections
    Meningitis
      Aseptic meningitis
      Meningitis; gram-negative (enteric/*Pseudomonas*)
      Meningitis; *Haemophilus influenzae*
      Meningitis; staphylococcal
      Meningitis; cryptococcal
      Meningitis; meningococcal
      Meningitis; pneumococcal
      Meningitis; tuberculous
    Subdural empyema
    Cavernous sinus thrombosis
  Tetanus
+Opportunistic infections
  +HIV infections
    AIDS (acquired immunodeficiency syndrome)
    Acute HIV infection
    Asymptomatic HIV infection
    Chronic symptomatic HIV infection (AIDS-related complex,
        ARC)
  AIDS-related Kaposi's sarcoma
  Atypical mycobacterial infection
  CMV (cytomegalovirus) gastroenteritis
  CMV in immunocompromised host

CMV pneumonia
CMV retinitis
Cryptosporidium enterocolitis
Disseminated tuberculosis
Esophagitis candida
Esophagitis CMV (cytomegalovirus)
Esophagitis herpes
Mucormycosis (zygomycosis)
Pneumocystis carinii pneumonia
Primary lymphoma of the brain
+Parasitic infections
  Ascariasis
  Cryptosporidium enterocolitis
  Echinococcosis
  Hookworm infection
  +Leishmoniasis
    Cutaneous leishmaniasis
    Visceral leishmaniasis
  Strongyloidosis
    Strongyloidosis; disseminated
  Malaria
  +Tapeworm infections
    Taenia saginata (beef tapeworm) infection
    Taenia solium (pork tapeworm) infection
      Cysticercosis
  Toxocariasis
  Toxoplasmosis in an immunocompromised host
  Trichinosis
+Sexually transmitted diseases
  Chancroid
  Chlamydia; female
  Chlamydial urethritis; male
  Gonococcemia (disseminated)
  Gonorrhea; female
  Gonorrhea; male
  Granuloma inguinale
  Herpes genital (genital herpes simplex)
  Lymphogranuloma venereum
  Neurosyphilis
  Syphilis; primary
  Syphilis; secondary
  Syphilis; tertiary
+Skin and soft tissue infections
  Carbunculosis or furunculosis
  Cat-scratch disease

Cellulitis
Cutaneous anthrax
Erysipelas
Erysipeloid
Folliculitis
Gas gangrene
Herpes simplex (herpes labialis)
Herpes zoster
Impetigo
Leprosy
Orf
Perianal abscess
Sporotrichosis
+URI upper respiratory infections
  Epiglottitis
  Gingivitis
  Otitis externa; acute
  Otitis externa; chronic
  Otitis externa; malignant
  Otitis media; acute
  Otitis media; chronic
  Parotitis
  Peritonsillar abscess (quinsy)
  Pharyngitis; gonococcal
  Pharyngitis; streptococcal
  Pharyngitis; viral
  Retropharyngeal abscess
  Sinusitis; acute
  Sinusitis; chronic
  Stomatitis, aphtous
+Vector-mediated diseases
  +Bacterial
    Lyme disease; primary
    Lyme disease; secondary
    Lyme disease; tertiary
    Plague
    Tularemia
  +Parasitic
    Malaria
  +Rickettsial
    Rocky Mountain spotted fever
    Typhus
  +Viral
    Colorado tick fever
    Yellow fever

    Hanta virus infection
+Viral infections NES (not elsewhere specified)
    Hand–foot–mouth disease
Herpangina
_____

+Miscellaneous
    Actinomycosis
    +Anthrax
        Cutaneous anthrax
        Inhalation anthrax
    Brucellosis
    Chlamydial pneumonia (psittacosis)
    +Conjunctivitis
    Legionella (Legionnaires' disease)
    Leptospirosis
    Nocardia infection
    Q fever (early)
    Q fever (late)
    Rat-bite fever
    Toxic shock syndrome
    Trachoma
    Typhoid fever
    Waterhouse–Friderichsen syndrome

+SPORTS MEDICINE

+Overuse (repetitive microtrauma) syndromes
    Achilles tendonitis
    Bicipital tendonitis
    Chondromalacia patellae
    ITB (iliotibial band) sydrome
    Lateral epicondylitis/tennis elbow
    Posterior tibial tendonitis
    Rotator cuff tendonitis
    Retrocalcaneal bursitis
    Stress fractures
+Acute injuries
    Ankle sprain
    Knee ligament injuries
        ACL (anterior cruciate ligament) injury
        PCL (posterior cruciate ligament) injury
        +MCL
            1st degree MCL (medial collateral ligament) injury
            2nd or 3rd degree MCL (medial collateral ligament) injury
        +LCL (lateral collateral ligament) injury

      1st degree LCL (lateral collateral ligament) injury
      2nd or 3rd degree LCL (lateral collateral ligament) injury
  Meniscus tears
  Muscle strain
  Patellar dislocation
  +Shoulder dislocation
      Shoulder dislocation/subluxation; acute anterior
      Shoulder dislocation/subluxation; recurrent anterior
      Shoulder dislocation/subluxation; acute posterior
      Shoulder dislocation/subluxation; recurrent posterior
      Shoulder dislocation/subluxation; multidirectional
  Shoulder separation
  Tendon rupture
  +Fractures
      Fracture of knee
      Fracture of ankle
      Fracture of shoulder
      Elbow, wrist, hands (metacarpals, phalanges)
      Feet (metatarsals, phalanges)

NEUROLOGICAL DISORDERS

  +Alcohol-related
      Alcohol withdrawal state
      Complicated alcohol abstinence (delirium tremens)
      Wernicke–Korsakoff syndrome
  +Dementia
      Chronic subdural hematoma
      Creutzfeldt–Jakob disease
      Dementia due to metabolic causes
      General paresis
      Huntington's disease
      Multi-infarct dementia
      Normal pressure hydrocephalus (NPH)
      Pick's disease
      Senile dementia/Alzheimer's type
      Subacute combined degeneration
      Wilson's disease
  +Demyelinating diseases
      Multiple sclerosis
        Optic neuritis
      Central pontine myelinolysis
      Progressive multifocal leukoencephalopathy
  +Headaches
      Classical migraine headache

    Common migraine headache
    Cluster headache
    Mixed tension migraine
    Tension headache
+Infectious
    Cerebral abscess
    Encephalitis (meningoencephalitis)
    +Meningitis
        Syphilitic aseptic meningitis
    Neurosyphilis
        Syphilitic myelopathy
        Tabes dorsalis
    Progressive multifocal leukoencephalopathy
+Inflammatory
    Bell's palsy
    Neurosarcoidosis
+Metabolic
    Hepatic encephalopathy
+Movement disorders
    +Drug-induced movement disorders
        Acute dystonic reaction
        Drug-induced parkinsonism
        Drug-induced tremor
        Tardive dyskinesia
    +Dystonia
        Idiopathic torsion dystonia
        +Focal dystonias
            Blepharospasm
            Occupational (writer's) cramp
            Oromandibular dystonia
            Spasmodic dysphonia
            Spasmodic torticollis (cervical dystonia)
        DOPA-responsive dystonia
    Essential tremor
        Familial tremor
    Friedreich's ataxia
    Huntington's disease
    +Multiple system atrophies
        Shy–Drager syndrome
        Striatonigral degeneration
        Olivopontocerebellar atrophy
    Parkinson's disease
    Progressive supranuclear palsy
    Stiff person syndrome
    +Tic disorders

      Gilles de la Tourette syndrome
      Chronic motor tic disorder
      Transient tic disorder
    Wilson's disease
+Myelopathies
    Amyotrophic lateral sclerosis
    Hereditary spastic paraplegia
    Myelopathy secondary to compression
    Subacute combined degeneration
    Syphilitic myelopathy
    Transverse myelitis
+Myopathies
    Becker's muscular dystrophy
    Dermatomyositis
    Duchenne's muscular dystrophy
    Facioscapulohumeral muscular dystrophy (Landousy–Dejerine)
    Familial periodic paralysis
    Hyperkalemic periodic paralysis (adynamia)
    Lambert–Eaton syndrome
    Limb-girdle muscular dystrophy
    Myasthenia gravis
    Myotonic dystrophy
    Polymyositis
    Thyrotoxic periodic paralysis
+Nervous system trauma
    Concussion
+Nervous system tumors
    Brain tumor—supratentorial
    Cerebellopontine angle tumor
    Metastatic brain tumor
    Pituitary tumor
    Primary brain tumor
    +Spinal cord tumor
      Cervical glioma
      Metastatic intraparenchymal spinal cord tumor
      Metastatic extraparenchymal spinal cord tumor
+Peripheral nerve diseases (lower motor neuron syndromes)
    +Motor neuron disease
      Amyotrophic lateral sclerosis
      Spinal muscular atrophy
    +Neuropathy
      +Mononeuropathy
        Axillary nerve dysfunction
        Common peroneal nerve dysfunction
        Distal median nerve dysfunction

Femoral nerve dysfunction
Radial nerve dysfunction
Sciatic nerve dysfunction
Ulnar nerve dysfunction
+Cranial neuropathies
  +Cranial nerve III neuropathy (oculomotor)
    Cranial mononeuropathy III; diabetic type
    Cranial mononeuropathy III; compression type
  Cranial mononeuropathy VI
  Cranial mononeuropathy VII
    Bell's palsy
Mononeuritis multiplex
+Polyneuropathy
  +Acute predominantly motor
    Guillain–Barre
    Paraneoplastic polyneuropathy
  +Subacute and chronic sensorimotor
    Alcoholic polyneuropathy
    Autonomic neuropathy
    Benign senile polyneuropathy
    Chronic inflammatory polyneuropathy
    Diabetic neuropathy
    +Hereditary motor and sensory polyneuropathy
      Charcot–Marie–Tooth disease
      Familial amyloid polyneuropathy
      Hereditary metabolic polyneuropathy
        (Refsum, Bassen-Kornzweig, Tangier, Fabry)
    Hypothyroid-related polyneuropathy
    Neuropathy secondary to drugs
    Toxic polyneuropathy
+Plexopathy
  Brachial plexopathy, unfinished
+Radiculopathy
  Cervical radiculopathy (C6/C7)
  Lumbar radiculopathy (S1)
+Paraneoplastic disorders (lung, breast, lymphoma)
  Cerebellar degeneration
  Dermatomyositis
  Lambert–Eaton syndrome
+Nerve distributions (i.e., neuropathies)
  Neuropathy secondary to drugs
+Seizure
  +Isolated seizure
    Febrile seizure
  Epilepsy

        Generalized tonic-clonic seizure (grand mal)
        Partial (focal) seizure
        Petit mal seizure
        Partial complex seizure
Stroke
    Hemorrhagic stroke
    Stroke secondary to atherosclerosis
    Stroke secondary to cardiogenic embolism
    Stroke secondary to carotid dissection
    Stroke secondary to carotid stenosis
    Stroke secondary to cocaine
    Stroke secondary to syphilis
    Transient ischemic attack (TIA)
+Intracranial hemorrhage
    Arteriovenous malformation (cerebral)
    Epidural hemorrhage
    +Hematoma
        Acute subdural hematoma
        Chronic subdural hematoma
    Subarachnoid hemorrhage (berry aneurysm)
    Intracerebral hemorrhage
        +Deep intracerebral hemorrhage
            Hypertensive intracerebral hemorrhage
        +Lobar intracerebral hemorrhage
            Senile cerebral amyloid angiopathy
        +Cortical
            Senile cerebral amyloid angiopathy
        Concussion
    Intraventricular hemorrhage (adult)
+Miscellaneous
    Pseudotumor cerebri
Cerebral palsy
    Neurofibromatosis-1
    Neurofibromatosis-2
    Tuberous sclerosis
+Sleep disorders
    +DIMS (disorder of initiating or maintaining sleep)
        +Breathing abnormalities
            Central sleep apnea
            Respiratory muscle weakness-associated sleep disorder
        +Drug-induced sleep disorders
            Stimulant-dependent sleep disorder
            Hypnotic-dependent sleep disorder
            Alcohol-dependent sleep disorder
        Natural short sleeper

    +Neurological abnormalities causing insomnia
      RLS (restless leg syndrome)
      Periodic limb movement disorder (PLMD)
    Psychophysiological (learned) insomnia
    +Sleep schedule disorder
      Chronic time zone change syndrome
      Shift work sleep disorder
      Irregular sleep-wake syndrome
      Delayed sleep phase syndrome
      Advanced sleep phase symdrome
      Non-24-hour sleep-wake disorder
    Sleep state misperception
  DOES (disorder of excessive sleepiness)
    Obstructive sleep apnea
    Narcolepsy
    Idiopathic hypersomnia
    +Sleep schedule disorder
      Chronic time zone change syndrome
      Shift work sleep disorder
      Irregular sleep-wake syndrome
      Delayed sleep phase syndrome
      Advanced sleep phase syndrome
      Non-24-hour sleep-wake disorder
    Central sleep apnea
  Parasomnia+
    REM-related+ (rapid eye movement)
      Repeated nightmares
      REM-behavior disorder
      Isolated sleep paralysis
    NREM-related+ (Non-REM)
      Night terror
      Nocturnal paroxysmal dystonia
      Sleep walking disorder (somnambulism)
      Sleep eating disorder

OPHTHALMOLOGIC DISORDERS

  +Cataract and other lens disorders
    Cataract (adult)
    Pediatric cataract
  +Cornea and external (conjunctival) disorders
    Blepharitis
      Blepharitis; allergic
      Blepharitis; atopic
      Blepharitis; staphylococcal

   Blepharitis; meibomitis
+Conjunctivitis
   Conjunctivitis; bacterial
   Conjunctivitis; viral
   Conjunctivitis; atopic
   Conjunctivitis; allergic
   Conjunctivitis; keratitis sicca
Corneal dysplasia/carcinoma
Corneal ulcer
+Keratoconus and other ectatic disorders
   Keratoconus
Pterygium
+Glaucoma
Glaucoma; acute angle closure
Glaucoma; open angle
Glaucoma; neovascular
+Neuro-ophthalmology
+Oculoplastics (lid, skin)
   Blepharospasm
   Chalazia
   Hordeolum
   Xanthelasma
+Retina and vitreal disorders
   +Age-related macular disease
      Macular degeneration
   Diabetic retinopathy with IDDM
   Diabetic retinopathy with NIDDM
   Hypertensive retinopathy
   Posterior vitreous detachment (floaters)
   Retinal detachment
   Retinitis pigmentosa
+Strabismus (eye motility disorders)
   Esotropia (crossed eyes)
   Exotropia (wall-eye)
   Hypertropia (vertical deviation of the eye)
   Paralytic heterotropia
+Trauma to the eye
   Hyphema
   Orbital blowout fracture
   Traumatic cataract
   Traumatic iritis
   Vitreous hemorrhage
+Uveitis
   Anterior uveitis
   Posterior uveitis

Panuveitis
+Visual disorders
    Amblyopia (lazy eye)
    Astigmatism
    Hyperopia (farsightedness)
    Myopia (nearsightedness)
    Presbyopia
Retinoblastoma

PEDIATRIC DISORDERS

+Behavioral and developmental pediatric disorders
    Attention deficit disorder (ADD)
    Autism
    Battered child syndrome
    Breath-holding spell
    Developmental delay
    Encopresis
    Precocious puberty
    +Sleep disorders
        Night terrors
        Nightmares
        Somnambulism
    Stuttering
+Cardiology
    ASD (atrial septal defect)
    Coarctation of aorta
    Kawasaki's disease
    Left-sided heart failure
    Rheumatic heart disease
    Tetralogy of Fallot
    VSD (ventricular septal defect)
+Dermatology
    Acne
    Acne neonatorum
    Alopecia areota
    Alopecia trichotillomania
    Cellulitis
    Diaper dermatitis; candida-associated
    Diaper dermatitis; irritant-induced
    Eczema
    Erythema toxicum
    Head lice (pediculosis capitis)
    Hemangioma
    Impetigo

Infant seborrheic dermatitis (cradle cap)
Milia
Miliaria crystallina
Miliaria rubra (prickly heat)
Nevus
Pityriasis rosea
Scabies
Sebaceous gland hyperplasia
Tinea
Traction alopecia
Urticaria
Wart, common
+Developmental
Communication disorder
Learning disorder
+EENT (eye-ear-nose-throat)
Acute sinusitis
Adenitis
Adenoid hypertrophy
Bacterial tracheitis
Branchial cleft cyst
Canker sore (aphthous ulcers)
Cerumen obstruction/impaction
Chronic sinusitis
Cystic hygroma
Epiglottitis
Epstein's pearls
Foreign body in the ear
Herpes gingivostomatitis
Nasal foreign body
Oral candidiasis (child)
Otitis externa
Otitis media
Otitis serous
Peritonsillar abscess
Retropharyngeal abscess
Pharyngitis, other
Rhinitis; acute
Rhinitis; allergic (hay fever)
Streptococcal pharyngitis
Thyroglossal duct cyst
Tonsillar hypertrophy
+Endocrine and metabolic
Acquired hypothyroidism
Adrenogenital disorder

Congenital hypothyroidism
Pediatric dehydration
+Short stature
  Constitutional growth delay
  Familial short stature
  Growth hormone deficiency
  Intrauterine growth retardation
  Malnutrition
  Nongrowth hormone-deficient short stature (Laron dwarfism)
  Psychosocial dwarfism
  Stimulant drugs
+Gastrointestinal system
  Anal fissure
  Anorexia nervosa
  +Bacterial enteritis
    Campylobacter enteritis
    E. coli enteritis
    Pseudomembranous colitis (*Clostridium difficile* enteritis)
    Salmonella enteritis
    Shigella enteritis
    Vibrio cholerae
    Yersinia enterocolitica
  Bulimia
  Childhood volvulus (midgut volvulus)
  Chronic dysfunctional stool retention
  Chronic recurrent abdominal pain (functional)
  Constipation
  Cow's milk or soy protein intolerance
  Cyclic vomiting
  Encopresis related to stool retention
  Entamoeba histolytica
  Idiopathic failure to thrive
  Food allergy
  Gastrointestinal foreign body
  Gastroesopohageal reflux (child)
  Gastroschisis
  Giardiasis
  Hirschsprung's disease
  Hypertrophic pyloric stenosis
  Infant colic
  Inguinal hernia
  Inguinal hernia (infant)
  Intussusception
  Lactase deficiency
    Postinfectious lactose intolerance
  Mallory–Weiss tear

Neonatal infections
  Neonatal hepatitis
  Neonatal *E. coli* sepsis
  TORCH syndrome (Toxoplasma Rubella CMV & Herpes
              Simplex mixed infection in the neonatal period)
  Neonatal UTI
+Newborn jaundice
  Physiological jaundice of the newborn
  Breast-milk jaundice
  +Hemolytic disease of the newborn
    ABO hemolytic disease of the newborn
    Rh hemolytic disease of the newborn
  Hyperbilirubinemia-associated upper intestinal obstruction
  Gilbert syndrome
  Crigler–Najjar syndrome
  Lucey–Driscoll syndrome
Omphalocele
Peptic ulcer
Swallowed blood
Tracheoesophageal fistula
Toddler's diarrhea
Umbilical hernia
Viral gastroenteritis
Viral hepatitis
Vomiting due to overfeeding
+Genetics/development
  Achondroplasia
  Down syndrome
  Fragile X syndrome
  Klinefelter's syndrome
  Neurofibromatosis I
  Niemann–Pick disease
  Osteogenesis imperfecta
  Pierre–Robin sequence
  Prader–Willi syndrome
  Spinal bifida
  Tay–Sachs disease
  Trisomy 13
  Trisomy 18
  Turner's syndrome
  Wilm's tumor
+Hematology
  Anemia
    Anemia of infection and chronic disease
    Aplastic and hypoplastic anemia
      Acquired aplastic anemia

      Congenital aplastic anemia
      Autoimmune hemolytic anemia
      Drug-induced immune hemolytic anemia
      Elliptocytosis
      Hemolytic disease of the newborn
        Erythroblastosis fetalis
      Hemolytic uremic syndrome
      Folate deficiency
      G6PD deficiency
      Hereditary spherocytosis
      Iron deficiency
      Methemoglobinemia
      Sickle cell disease
      Thalassemia
        α-Thalassemia
        Heterozygous beta-thalassemia (beta-thalassemia trait)
        Homozygous beta-thalassemia (beta-thalassemia major)
      Vitamin B_{12} deficiency
+Infectious disease
    Chicken pox
    Pinworms
    Erythema infectiosum
    Roseola
    Hand-foot-and-mouth disease
    Herpangina
    Acute mastoiditis
    Measles (rubeola)
    Mononucleosis
    Mumps
    +Neonatal infections
      CMV
      Congenital rubella (German measles)
      Hepatitis
      Herpes simplex virus
      Neonatal group B strep infection; early-onset
      Neonatal group B strep infection; late-onset
      Neonatal HIV
      Syphilis
      Toxoplasmosis
      Varicella
    Rabies
    Rubella (German measles)
    Scalded skin syndrome
    Scarlatina
    Vaccine reaction

Vulvovaginitis (yeast, monoliasis)??
Whooping cough (pertussis)
+Musculoskeletal
  Clubfoot
  Congenital hip dysplasia
  Congenital torticollis
  Craniosynostosis
  Discitis
  Ingrown toenail
  Kawasaki's disease
  Legg–Calve–Perthes disease
  Neonatal clavicular fracture
  Nursemaid's elbow
  Osgood–Schlatter disease
  Slipped capital femoral epiphysis
  +Torsional deformity
    Adducted great toe
    Metatarsus adductus
    Medial tibial torsion
    Medial femoral torsion
  Toxic synovitis
+Neurological
  Aseptic meningitis
  Cerebral palsy
  Febrile seizure
  Head injury, closed
  Headache
  +Hypotonia
    Central hypotonia
    Spinal muscular atrophy type I (Werdnig–Hoffman disease)
    Spinal muscular atrophy type II intermediate type
    Spinal muscular atrophy juvenile type (Kugelberg–Welander
        disease)
    Infant botulism
  Intraventricular hemorrhage (IVH)
  Meningitis, bacterial
  Migraine headache
  Neuroblastoma
  Pseudotumor cerebri in an infant
  Seizure
  Tension headache
+Ophthalmology
  +Acute conjunctivitis
    Conjunctivitis; bacterial
    Conjunctivitis; viral

    Conjunctivitis; atopic
    Conjunctivitis; vernal
  Color blindness
  Corneal abrasion
  Dacryostenosis
  +Ophthalmia neonatorum
    Ophthalmia neonatorum; *Chlamydia*-associated
    Ophthalmia neonatorum; gonorrhea-associated
  Orbital cellulitis
  Pediatric cataract
  Periorbital cellulitis
  +Strabismus
    Esotropia
    Exotropia
+Pulmonary
  Apnea
  Pediatric asthma
  Bronchopulmonary dysplasia
  Bronchiolitis
  Croup (laryngotracheitis)
    Spasmodic croup
  +Neonatal respiratory distress syndromes
    Neonatal respiratory distress syndrome (NRDS)
  Pediatric pneumonia
  Pneumonia
  Tracheal or bronchial foreign body
+Renal and urology
  Cystitis
  Dehydration
    Hypotonic dehydration
    Hypertonic dehydration
    Isotonic dehydration
  Enuresis
  Hydrocele
  Hydronephrosis
  Hypertension
  Hypospadius
  Meatal stenosis
  Pyelonephritis
  Undescended testes
  Urethritis
  Vesicoureteral reflux
  Wilm's tumor
+Toxicology
  Lead poisoning
  Aspirin poisoning

    Acetaminophen poisoning
+Miscellaneous
    Reye's syndrome

PSYCHIATRIC DISORDERS

+Affective disorders (mood disorders)
    +Major depressive episode (acute depression) (unipolar)
        Major depression
            Major depression with psychotic features
    Neurotic depression (dysthymia)
    +Bipolar disorder
        Bipolar disorder (manic)
        Bipolar disorder (depressed)
    Seasonal affect disorder
+Adjustment disorder
    Adjustment disorder with depressed mood
    Adjustment disorder with anxious mood
    Adjustment disorder with mixed emotional features
+Anxiety disorders
    Generalized anxiety disorder
    Obsessive-compulsive disorder
    Panic disorder
    Posttraumatic stress disorder
    Simple phobia
    Social phobia
At risk for suicide
+Cognitive disorders
    Alzheimer's cognitive disorder
    Schizophrenia; paranoid
    Schizophrenia; undifferentiated
    Schizophrenia; disorganized (hebephrenic)
    Schizoaffective disorder
+Organic mental disorder
    Organic mood disorder
    Organic psychotic disorder
+Personality disorders
    +Personality disorder—A (odd/eccentric)
        Personality disorder; paranoid
        Personality disorder; schizoid
        Personality disorder; schizotypal
    +Personality disorder—B (dramatic, emotional, erratic)
        Personality disorder; histrionic
        Personality disorder; antisocial
        Personality disorder; narcissistic
        Personality disorder; borderline

+Personality disorder—C (anxious/fearful)
  Personality disorder; avoidant
  Personality disorder; dependent
  Personality disorder; obsessive/compulsive
  Personality disorder; passive-aggressive
+Somatoform disorders
  Conversion disorder
  Hypochondriasis
  Somatization disorder
  Somatoform pain disorder
+Somatoform-related disorders
  Malingering
    Factitious disorder with physical symptoms
    Factitious disorder with psychological symptoms
+Substance abuse
  Alcohol dependence (alcoholism)
  Alcohol- or drug-induced psychosis
  Amphetamine/sympathomimetic intoxication
  Barbiturate intoxication
  Caffeine intoxication
  Cannabis intoxication
  Cocaine intoxication
  Cocaine withdrawal
  Nicotine withdrawal
  Opioid withdrawal
  Opioid intoxication
+Miscellaneous
  Noncompliance
  Brief reactive psychosis
  Compulsive gambling
  Depression in the elderly
+Pediatric psychiatric disorders
  +Childhood mood disorders
    Childhood depression
  +Disruptive behavior disorders
    Attention deficit disorder
    Conduct disorder
    Oppositional defiant disorder
  +Pervasive developmental disorder
    Asperger's disorder
    Autism
    Childhood disintegrative disorder
    Mental retardation
    Rett's syndrome
  Mental retardation

+Elimination disorders
  Encopresis
  Enuresis
Separation anxiety
+Sexual dysfunction
  Hypoactive sexual desire
  Sexual aversion disorder
  Female sexual arousal disorder
  Male erectile disorder (psychogenic)
  Female orgasmic disorder (psychogenic)
  Male orgasmic disorder (psychogenic)
  Drug-induced excessive penile erection
  Dyspareunia (psychogenic)
  Vaginismus (psychogenic)

RESPIRATORY DISORDERS

+Diaphragmatic diseases
  Diaphragm paralysis (unilateral)
  Diaphragm paralysis (bilateral)
+Environmental and occupational lung diseases
  Acute chemical pulmonary injury
  Acute mountain sickness
    HIgh-altitude cerebral edema
    High-altitude pulmonary edema
  Drug-induced pulmonary disease
  Hypersensitivity pneumonitis (allergic alveolitis)
  Industrial bronchitis
  +Pneumoconiosis (silicosis, asbestos, coal, etc.)
    Asbestosis
    Asbestos-related pleural calcification
    Asbestos-related pleural fibrosis
    Asbestos-related pleural effusion
    Coal workers' pneumoconiosis
    Silicosis (classical)
    Silicosis; acute
      Caplan's syndrome (rheumatoid pneumoconiosis)
    Berylliosis
  Occupational asthma
  Silo filler's disease
+Infectious diseases of the lung
  +Pneumonias; bacterial
    Hospital-acquired pneumonia
    Pneumonia
    Pneumonia in immunocompromised host

Necrotizing pneumonia (pneumonia with lung abscess)
Mycoplasma pneumonia
Chlamydial pneumonia (psittacosis)
Legionella (Legionnaire's disease)
+Pneumonias; viral
  Influenza
  Viral pneumonia
+Mycobacterial diseases
  Atypical mycobacterial infection
  Disseminated tuberculosis
  Pulmonary tuberculosis
+Fungal diseases of the lung
  Blastomycosis
  Coccidiomycosis; acute (primary) pulmonary
  Coccidiomycosis; disseminated
  Coccidiomycosis; chronic pulmonary
  Histoplasmosis; acute (primary) pulmonary
  Histoplasmosis; disseminated (acute)
  Histoplasmosis; chronic pulmonary
  Pulmonary actinomycosis
  Pulmonary aspergillosus; invasive type
  Pulmonary aspergillosus; allergic bronchopulmonary type
  Pulmonary aspergilloma (mycetoma)
  Pulmonary nocardiosis
+Parasitic lung diseases
  Echinococcus
+Infiltrative and interstitial lung diseases
  +Connective tissue disorders
    Lymphomatoid granulomatosis
    Rheumatoid lung disease
    Pulmonary scleroderma
    Pulmonary systemic lupus erythematosus
    Wegener's granulomatosis
  Diffuse interstitial pulmonary fibrosis
    Idiopathic diffuse interstitial pulmonary fibrosis
  Pulmonary alveolar proteinosis
  Sarcoidosis
  +Pulmonary hemosiderosis
    Goodpasture's syndrome
    Idiopathic pulmonary hemosiderosis (adult)
    Pulmonary lymphangioleiomyomatosis
  +Eosinophilic syndromes
    Acute pulmonary eosinophilia (Loeffler's syndrome)
    Chronic eosinophilic pneumonia
    Pulmonary histiocytosis X (eosinophilic granuloma)
+Mediastinal diseases

   Acute mediastinitis
   Mediastinal fibrosis (granulomatous mediastinitis)
   Mediastinal emphysema (pneumomediastinum)
+Neoplasms of the lung
   Primary lung cancer
   Metastatic cancer to the lung
   Solitary pulmonary nodule (benign)
   Solitary pulmonary nodule (malignant)
   Bronchial adenoma
      Bronchial carcinoid
   Mesothelioma (malignant)
+Obstructive airway disease
   Acute upper airway obstruction
   Bronchial asthma
   Bronchiectasis
   Emphysema
      Alpha-1-antitrypsin deficiency
      Giant bullous emphysema
   Acute bronchitis
   Bronchiolitis obliterans with organizing pneumonia (BOOP)
   Bronchiolitis obliterans without organizing pneumonia
   Chronic bronchitis
   Cystic fibrosis
+Pleural diseases
   +Pleural effusion
      +Exudative pleural effusion
         Parapneumonic pleural effusion
         Rheumatoid pleural effusion
         Tuberculous pleural effusion
      Transudative pleural effusion
   Chylothorax
   Empyema
   +Pneumothorax
      Spontaneous pneumothorax
      Traumatic pneumothorax
      Tension pneumothorax
   +Tumors of the pleura
      Mesothelioma (malignant)
      Mesothelioma (benign-fibrous)
      Metastatic pleural tumor
   Fibrothorax
   Hemothorax
+Respiratory insufficiency
   ARDS (adult respiratory distress syndrome)
   Chronic respiratory failure
   +Disorders in the control of breathing

       Chemically induced alveolar hypoventilation
       Obesity hypoventilation syndrome (Pickwickian syndrome)
       Obstructive sleep apnea
   +Disorders of the chest wall
       Fibrothorax
       Flail chest
       Kyphoscoliosis lung disease
  +Vascular intrathoracic disorders
    +Thromboembolism
       Pulmonary embolus
    +Pulmonary hypertension
       Primary pulmonary hypertension
       Pulmonary AV fistula
       Pulmonary venoocclusive disease
       Cor pulmonale

RENAL AND UROLOGICAL DISORDERS

  Acute nephritic syndrome
    +Primary renal
       Poststreptococcal glomerulonephritis (GN)
       IgA nephropathy (Berger's disease)
       Membranoproliferative GN I
       Membranoproliferative GN II
       IgM mesangial proliferative glomerulonephritis
    +Secondary causes
       Henoch–Schonlein
       Hemolytic uremic syndrome (HUS)
       Lupus nephritis
       Rapidly progressive (crescentic) glomerulonephritis
         +Type I (Anti-GBM nephritis) (glomerular basement
             membrane)
          Goodpasture's disease
         +Type II (immune complex disease)
         +Type III (pauci-immune disease)
          Wegener's disease
          Microscopic polyarteritis
  Acute renal failure
    Acute interstitial nephritis caused by NSAIDs (nonsteroidal
             antiinflammatory drugs)
    Acute interstitial nephritis not NSAID-related
    Acute tubular necrosis
       Rhabdomyolysis
    Hemodynamically induced renal failure
    Hepatorenal syndrome

Prerenal azotemia
Scleroderma renal crisis
Chronic renal failure
  Chronic glomerulonephritis
  End-stage renal disease
+Cystic renal diseases
  Acquired cystic disease
  Medullary cystic disease
  Polycystic kidney disease
+Drug-induced renal dysfunction
+Fluid and electrolyte imbalance
  +Diabetes insipidus; nephrogenic
    Diabetes insipidus; nephrogenic (acquired)
    Diabetes insipidus; nephrogenic (congenital)
  Renal tubular acidosis; distal (type I)
  Renal tubular acidosis; proximal (type II)
  Renal tubular acidosis; type IV
  Hyperkalemia may be due to a drug
  Hyperkalemia
  Hypokalemia
  Hypernatremia
  Hyponatremia
  Hypophosphatemia
  Hyperphosphatemia
  Hypercalcemia
  Hypocalcemia
+Hereditary renal diseases
  Alport syndrome
+Hypertension
  Essential hypertension
  +Secondary hypertension
    Renovascular hypertension (renal artery stenosis)
  Malignant hypertension (arteriolar nephrosclerosis)
+Interstitial nephritis
  Acute interstitial nephritis caused by NSAIDs
  Acute interstitial nephritis not NSAID-related
  Analgesic nephropathy
  Hemodynamically induced renal failure
  Reflux nephropathy
  Renal papillary necrosis
+Metabolic nephropathy
  Uric acid nephropathy, acute
  Uric acid nephropathy, chronic (gouty nephropathy)
Nephrotic syndrome
  Diabetic nephropathy/sclerosis

Focal segmental glomerulosclerosis
Lupus nephritis
Membranous nephropathy
Minimal change disease
+Obstructive renal disease
  Acute bilateral obstructive uropathy
  Acute unilateral obstructive uropathy
  Chronic bilateral obstructive uropathy
  Chronic unilateral obstructive uropathy
    Ureterocele
  Nephrolithiasis
    Calcium oxalate calculi
    Struvite calculi ($MgNH_4PO_4$, infection stones)
    Cystinuria
    Uric acid calculi
  Retroperitoneal fibrosis
+Renal and urinary tract tumors
  Carcinoma of the renal pelvis or ureter
  Renal cell carcinoma (hypernephroma)
  Transitional cell carcinoma of the bladder
+Renovascular abnormalities
  Atheroembolic renal disease
  HUS
  Renal artery stenosis
  Renal vein thrombosis
  Scleroderma renal crisis
+UTI (urinary tract infection)
  Acute uncomplicated pyelonephritis
  Asymptomatic bacteriuria
  Catheter-associated UTI
  Complicated UTI ("chronic pyelonephritis")
  +Cystitis
    Cystitis; acute bacterial (uncomplicated UTI)
    Cystitis; interstitial (Hunner's ulcer)
    Cystitis; noninfectious (acute urethral syndrome)
    Cystitis; recurrent
  Tuberculous renal disease
  Epididymitis
+Renal tumors
  Carcinoma of the urinary bladder
  Wilm's tumor
+Miscellaneous
  Ruptured abdominal aortic aneurysm
+Prostatic diseases
  Prostatitis; acute
  Prostatitis; chronic

Prostatitis; nonbacterial
Benign prostatic hyperplasia
Prostatic cancer
+Scrotal diseases
Testicular torsion
Hydrocele
Varicocele
+Testicular tumor
Seminoma
Nonseminoma testicular tumor

RHEUMATOLOGICAL DISORDERS

+Inflammatory
+Connective tissue disease
Adult Still's
Behcet's syndrome
Dermatomyositis
Eosinophilic fasciitis
Giant cell (temporal; cranial) arteritis
Henoch–Schonlein purpura
Necrotizing vasculitis
+Juvenile RA (rheumatoid arthritis)
Juvenile RA; systemic onset
Juvenile RA; polyarticular onset
Juvenile RA; pauciarticular onset
Polymyalgia rheumatica
Polymyositis (adult)
Relapsing polychondritis
Rheumatoid arthritis
Felty's syndrome
Sjogren syndrome
Systemic lupus erythematosus
Drug-induced lupus erythematosus
Systemic sclerosis (scleroderma)
CREST syndrome (calcinosis cutis, Raynaud's syndrome,
esophageal dysfunction, sclerodactyly,
telangiectasia)
Raynaud's phenomenon
+Reactive arthritis
Ankylosing spondylitis
Enteropathic arthropathy
Psoriatic arthritis
Reiter's syndrome
Rheumatic fever; adult
Rheumatic fever; child

+Crystal-induced
  +Gout
    Acute gouty arthritis
    Chronic gouty arthritis
  Pseudogout
+Degenerative
  Chondromalacia patellae
  Neuropathic joint disease (Charcot joint)
  Osteoarthritis
+Infectious
  +Fungal arthritis
    Fungal arthritis; blastomycotic
    Fungal arthritis; *Candida*
    Fungal arthritis; coccidiodal
    Fungal arthritis; sporotrichosis
  Gonococcal arthritis
  Nongonococcal (septic) bacterial arthritis
  Osteomyelitis
  Tuberculous arthritis
  Viral arthritis
+Soft tissue
  Adhesive capsulitis
  Bicipital tendonitis
  Bursitis
  Calcific tendonitis
  Carpal tunnel syndrome
  Fibrositis (fibromyalgia)
  Lateral epicondylitis/tennis elbow
  Rotator cuff tendinitis
+Back pain
  Compression fractures of the back
  Herniated nucleus pulposus (slipped disk)
  Nonspecific back pain
  Spinal stenosis
+Genetic musculoskeletal disorders
  Marfan's syndrome
  Ehlers–Danlos syndrome (type unspecified)
  Osteogenesis imperfecta (type unspecified)

+Miscellaneous rheumatological diseases
  Avascular (aseptic) necrosis
  Hypertrophic osteoarthropathy
  Paget's disease
  Reflex sympathetic dystrophy

Appendix 2
Approximate Estimated Prevalences for Selected Top-Level Diseases in a Family Practice Setting, Categorized by Specialty

Note that some a prioris vary markedly by geographical location. This list was compiled for use in the Salt Lake City, UT, area. The population is assumed to be 30% pediatric. Although almost all patients will have some skin lesion, it is assumed that only 30% of the time a skin lesion will be included in the patients' diseases; this also applies for mild psychiatric illnesses and some chronic diseases. Only the first visit for a given problem contributes to the statistic. Well-baby checkups, or other health maintenance visits, would not be included in the total. The reliability of the numbers varies from very certain to very uncertain.

CARDIOVASCULAR DISEASES

Acute MI (myocardial infarct)	.01
Alcoholic cardiomyopathy	.002
Angiosarcoma	.00001
Aortic dissection	.00015
Aortic insufficiency	.0013
Aortic stenosis	.002
Arteriosclerosis obliterans (peripheral vascular disease)	.002
Atrial fibrillation/flutter	.02
Atrial myxoma; left	.00004
Atrial myxoma; right	.000005
Atrial septal defect	.0004
AV (atrioventricular) block (2nd or 3rd degree)	.0005
Carcinoid heart disease	.000001
Cardiac tamponade	.001
Chagas' disease	.000001
Chest wall pain	.005
Chronic venous insufficiency	.015
Coarctation of the aorta	.0001

Coronary artery spasm	.0002
Cystic hygroma	.0001
Deep venous thrombophlebitis of extremity	.015
Digitalis toxicity	.001
Dilated cardiomyopathy	.02
Echocardiographic findings of cardiac tamponade	.001
Essential hypertension	.25
Hypertensive heart disease	.03
Hypertrophic cardiomyopathy	.0001
Hypovolemia	.004
Ischemic cardiomyopathy	.02
Klippel–Trenaunay syndrome	.00001
Left ventricular enlargement	.06
Left-sided heart failure	.02
Low cardiac output	.025
Lymphangioma	.00001
Lymphedema; primary	.003
Lymphedema; secondary	.0065
Mitral regurgitation; acute	.0005
Mitral regurgitation; chronic (mitral insufficiency)	.005
Mitral stenosis	.001
Mitral valve prolapse	.002
Multifocal atrial tachycardia (MAT)	.003
Myocardial contusion	.00001
Myocarditis	.0001
Paroxysmal supraventricular tachycardia (PSVT)	.01
Pelvic vein thrombophlebitis	.0015
Pericarditis	.003
Pericarditis; bacterial	.00012
Pericarditis; postmyocardial infarction (Dressler's)	.0005
Peripartum cardiomyopathy	.0004
Peripheral arterial embolism	.001
Postphlebitic syndrome	.0025
Pulmonary venous congestion	.025
Restrictive cardiomyopathy	.001
Right-sided heart failure	.01
Risk factors for peripheral vascular disease	.20
Risk of atherosclerosis	.20
Risk of thrombophlebitis	.15
Ruptured abdominal aortic aneurysm	.0005
Sick sinus syndrome	.0006
Stable angina	.035
Superficial thrombophlebitis of extremity	.02
Thromboangiitis obliterans (Buerger's disease)	.0006
Tricuspid regurgitation	.003

Unstable angina	.02
Varicose vein(s); primary	.0075
Varicose vein(s); secondary	.005
Venous incompetence	.009
Ventricular tachycardia	.001
Wolff–Parkinson–White syndrome	.0015

DERMATOLOGIC DISEASES

Acanthosis nigricans	.0005
Acne	.15
Actinic keratosis	.05
Allergic vasculitis	.00025
Angioedema	.005
Atopic dermatitis	.01
Bacterial paronychia	.0005
Basal cell carcinoma	.0025
Basal cell carcinoma; morpheaform	.000125
Body lice (pediculosis corporis)	.00005
Bullous ichthyosiform erythroderma (epidermolytic hyperkeratosis)	.000005
Bullous pemphigoid	.0005
Candida paronychia	.0005
Condyloma (genital wart)	.01
Contact dermatitis	.01
Cutaneous candidiasis	.005
Cutaneous cyst	.004
Darier's disease (keratosis follicularis)	.00006
Dermatofibroma	.005
Discoid lupus erythematosus	.002
Dyshidrotic eczema	.02
EB (epidermolysis bullosa) dystrophic	.000003
EB junctional	.0000007
EB simplex	.000028
Erythema marginatum	.00001
Erythema multiforme	.001
Folliculitis decalvans	.00001
Gottron's papule	.00007
Granuloma annulare	.0006
Grover's disease (transient acantholytic dermatosis)	.0001
Hereditary hemorrhagic telangiectasia (Osler–Weber–Rendu)	.0001
Ichthyosis vulgaris	.004
Insect bite	.005
Keloid	.0005

Keratoacanthoma	.001
Kerion	.00001
Lamellar ichthyosis	.000004
Lesion of guttate psoriasis	.003
Lichen planopilaris	.00001
Lichen planus	.001
Lichen simplex chronicus	.005
Melasma	.001
Molluscum contagiosum	.0004
Mycosis fungoides (cutaneous T-cell lymphoma)	.00001
Nummular eczema	.02
Orf	.00001
Pemphigus vulgaris	.0001
Pityriasis rosea	.0035
Porphyria cutanea tarda	.0001
Psoriasis; guttate	.003
Pubic lice (pediculosis pubis)	.001
Rosacea	.01
Scabies	.0025
Scaly or hyperkeratotic macule	.02
Seborrheic dermatitis	.02
Seborrheic keratosis	.01
Skin findings of neurofibromatosis	.0001
Skin tag (acrochordon)	.02
Solitary neurofibroma	.0001
Spider bite	.001
Squamous cell carcinoma	.0005
Stasis dermatitis	.005
Superficial spreading melanoma	.0002
Tinea capitis	.001
Tinea corporis	.005
Tinea pedis	.025
Tinea versicolor	.005
Urticaria	.01
Vitiligo	.004
Wart	.008
Xerosis	.04

ENDOCRINE AND METABOLIC DISEASES

Acromegaly	.00006
Acute adrenal crisis	.00002
Addison's disease	.00005
Adrenal apoplexy	.000012
Adrenal insufficiency	.00025

Adrenoleukodystrophy .000001
Alcoholic ketoacidosis .0001
Anaplastic carcinoma of the thyroid .0003
Anorexia nervosa .0012
Autoimmune ovarian failure .0005
Bartter's syndrome .000005
Benign prostatic hyperplasia .05
Bulimia .004
CAH (female; classical) (chronically active hepatitis) .0002
CAH (female; nonclassical) .003
Carcinoid syndrome .000025
Chronic thyroiditis (Hashimoto's disease) .01
Chylomicronemia syndrome .0005
Clinical manifestations of hypometabolism .01
Colloid nodular goiter .02
Congenital lipodystrophy .000001
Craniopharyngioma .0005
Cushing's syndrome caused by adrenal tumor .000006
Cushing's syndrome; endogenous .0002
Cushing's syndrome; exogenous .0005
Cystathionine beta-synthetase deficiency .000003
Cystinosis .000004
Cystinuria .00005
Diabetes insipidus .0002
Diabetic hyperglycemic hyperosmolar coma .0002
Diabetic ketoacidosis .001
Drug-induced hypoglycemia .009
Drug-induced hypothyroidism .0002
Ectopic Cushing's syndrome .000004
Ectopic SIADH .0005
Empty sella syndrome .00001
Episodes suggesting catecholamine excess .01
Ethylene glycol intoxication .00005
Euthyroid sick syndrome .005
Exogenous adrenal insufficiency .005
Fabry's disease .000025
Facticious hyperthyroidism .00002
Facticious hypoglycemia .0001
Familial combined hyperlipidemia .005
Familial dysbetalipoproteinemia .0001
Familial hypercholesterolemia .002
Familial hypertriglyceridemia .002
Familial lipoprotein lipase deficiency .000001
Familial Mediterranean fever .000005
Familial periodic paralysis .00001

Fanconi's syndrome; acquired	.00002
Fanconi's syndrome; familial	.000001
Folate deficiency	.001
Follicular tumor of the thyroid (adenoma or carcinoma)	.001
Fructose intolerance	.00005
Fructose-1,6-diphosphatase deficiency	.000001
Galactosemia (due to kinase deficiency)	.00002
Galactosemia (due to transferase deficiency)	.00002
Gastrinoma (Zollinger–Ellison syndrome)	.000056
Glucagonoma	.000001
Graves' disease	.001
Hemochromatosis	.0015
Hereditary amyloidosis	.000005
Hereditary urea cycle abnormality	.000001
Hormone-induced hypercalcemia	.003
Hypercalcemia	.005
Hypercalcemia of malignancy	.0003
Hyperkalemic periodic paralysis (adynamia)	.00001
Hyperlipidemia pattern of CAD (coronary artery disease)	.20
Hyperlipidemia pattern of pancreatitis	.001
Hyperlipidemia; acquired	.05
Hyperornithinemia	.000001
Hyperthyroidism	.003
Hyperthyroxinemia without hyperthyroidism	.0001
Hypertriglyceridemia; sporadic	.03
Hypoglycemia	.01
Hypogonadotrophic hypogonadism (Kallman's syndrome)	.00005
Hypomagnesemia	.001
Hypomagnesemia	.001
Hypoparathyroidism	.0001
Hypophosphatemia	.001
Hypopituitarism	.00015
Hyporeninemic hypoaldosteronism	.0001
Hypothyroidism	.022
Hypothyroidism; primary	.01
Hypothyroidism; secondary	.002
IDDM (insulin-dependent diabetes mellitus)	.008
Idiopathic hypercalciuria	.005
Insulinoma	.00001
Ketoacidosis	.001
Klinefelter's syndrome	.001
Leydig cell tumor	.000001
Malnutrition	.01

Maple syrup urine disease	.000005
McArdle's syndrome (glycogen storage disease type V)	.000005
Medullary carcinoma of thyroid	.0004
MEN I (multiple endocrine neoplasias)	.00001
MEN II	.00003
Methanol intoxication	.0001
Mild secondary hyperparathyroidism	.001
Milk-alkali syndrome	.0001
Myxedema coma	.000001
Narcolepsy	.0003
Nelson's syndrome	.0000001
NIDDM (non-insulin-dependent diabetes mellitus)	.03
Nonfunctional benign adrenal mass	.01
Nonseminoma testicular tumor	.00005
Oncogenic osteomalacia	.00001
Osteomalacia	.001
Osteoporosis (symptomatic)	.03
Painless (silent) thyroiditis	.0002
Papillary carcinoma of the thyroid	.006
Pellagra (niacin deficiency)	.00001
Pheochromocytoma	.0001
Pituitary adrenal insufficiency	.00003
Pituitary Cushing's (Cushing's disease)	.00003
Polycystic ovary syndrome	.001
Polygenic hypercholesterolemia	.02
Primary hyperaldosteronism	.00002
Primary hyperparathyroidism	.001
Prolactinome, females	.001
Prolactinoma, males	.0003
Prostatic cancer	.001
Pseudohypoparathyroidism	.00005
Pyridoxine (vitamin B_6) deficiency	.00001
Rickets	.001
Salt-losing congenital adrenal hyperplasia	.00004
Scurvy	.0001
Seminoma	.00002
Severe secondary hyperparathyroidism	.0001
SIADH (dilutional hyponatremia)	.005
Signs and symptoms of cachexia or marasmus	.01
Signs and symptoms of sympathetic hyperactivity	.01
Signs of ketoacidosis	.00225
Subacute thyroiditis	.0001
Testosterone-producing adrenal adenoma	.000001
Thiamine deficiency (beriberi)	.0005
Thyroid hemorrhage	.00001

Thyroid lymphoma   .0001
Thyrotoxic storm   .000004
Toxic nodular goiter   .0003
Turner's syndrome   .001
Vitamin A deficiency   .0001
Vitamin A toxicity   .000001
Vitamin B_2 deficiency   .0001
Vitamin D toxicity   .00003
Vitamin K deficiency   .005
Vitamin K deficiency   .005
Von Gierke's disease   .00002

GASTROINTESTINAL DISEASES

Achalasia   .0005
Acute appendicitis   .0005
Acute cholangitis   .0001
Acute cholecystitis   .003
Acute colonic pseudo-obstruction (Ogilivie's syndrome)   .0001
Acute pancreatitis   .001
Adenocarcinoma of the small bowel   .00001
Adenomatous small bowel polyp   .00002
Alcoholic liver disease (hepatitis/cirrhosis)   .001
Amebiasis   .00001
Amebic liver abscess   .000001
Angiodysplasia of the GI tract   .0005
Ascites   .005
Autoimmune hepatitis   .0004
Bacterial gastroenteritis   .002
Bile salt malabsorption   .001
Biliary obstruction   .005
Biliary pain   .01
Biliary stricture   .0002
Bleeding esophageal varices   .001
Campylobacter enteritis   .0005
Celiac disease (sprue)   .00025
Cholangiocarcinoma   .00005
Choledocholithiasis   .0002
Cholelithiasis   .0029
Cholera   .00001
Cholestatic jaundice   .01
Chronic active hepatitis   .00012
Chronic autoimmune gastritis (atrophic gastritis)   .0004
Chronic cholecystitis   .0028
Chronic cholecystitis; acute episode   .0028

Chronic intestinal pseudo-obstruction	.00001
Chronic pancreatitis	.0003
Chronic persistent hepatitis	.0006
Cirrhosis	.002
Colon cancer	.001
Colorectal polyps ≥1 cm	.02
Crigler–Najjar disease; type I	.000001
Crigler–Najjar disease; type II	.00002
Crohn's disease; regional enteritis	.002
Delta agent (hepatitis D)	.000008
Diverticular colonic bleed	.0005
Diverticulitis	.0035
Diverticulosis	.05
Drug-induced cholestasis	.0001
Drug-induced diarrhea	.005
Drug-induced hepatitis	.0005
Duodenal ulcer	.0056
E. coli enteritis	.0003
Esophageal cancer	.0005
Esophageal perforation	.0001
Esophageal spasm	.001
Esophageal stricture (benign)	.0015
Familial adenomatous polyposis	.001
Fatty liver of pregnancy	.000001
Fecal impaction	.001
Gastric cancer	.0008
Gastric outlet obstruction	.00024
Gastric ulcer; benign	.003
Gastritis; acute	.001
Gastroesophageal reflux disease	.01
Gastrointestinal manifestations of non-Hodgkin's lymphoma	.00002
Gastrointestinal perforation	.0001
Gastroparesis	.002
Giant hypertrophic gastritis (Menetrier's disease)	.00005
Giardiasis	.001
Gilbert's syndrome	.05
Helicobacter pylori gastritis (chronic gastritis)	.01
Hemorrhoids	.10
Hepatic encephalopathy	.0004
Hepatic focal nodular hyperplasia	.00001
Hepatic hemangioma	.0004
Hepatic vein obstruction (Budd–Chiari)	.00001
Hepatitis A	.0004
Hepatitis B	.0008

Hepatitis C	.0008
Hepatocellular adenoma	.00002
Hepatocellular carcinoma	.0004
Hepatocellular jaundice	.01
High risk factors for hepatitis B	.001
Intestinal bacterial overgrowth (blind loop syndrome)	.0001
Intestinal leiomyoma	.00002
Intestinal lymphangiectasia	.0003
Intestinal lymphatic obstruction	.00006
Intestinal obstruction	.001
Intestinal volvulus	.0001
Intraabdominal abscess	.0005
Intrahepatic cholestasis of pregnancy	.0001
Irritable bowel syndrome (functional bowel)	.007
Ischemic colitis	.0003
Ischemic hepatocellular jaundice	.0005
Lactase deficiency	.01
Liver metastases	.001
Lower esophageal ring (Schatzki's)	.001
Malabsorption	.002
Mallory–Weiss tear	.0008
Meckel's diverticulum	.0001
Nonalcoholic steatohepatitis	.0001
Pain of esophageal spasm	.001
Pancreas divisum	.01
Pancreatic abscess	.0002
Pancreatic carcinoma	.0006
Pancreatic pseudocyst	.001
Peliosis hepatis	.0001
Physical findings of Crohn's disease	.01
Pneumatosis cystoides intestinalis	.0001
Polycystic liver disease	.0002
Portal hypertension	.005
Postnecrotic cirrhosis	.00008
Primary biliary cirrhosis	.00005
Protein-losing gastroenteropathy	.0001
Pseudomembranous colitis	.0005
Pyogenic liver abscess	.00001
Radiation enteritis	.00006
Salmonella enteritis	.0005
Sclerosing cholangitis	.0001
Shigella enteritis	.0002
Short bowel syndrome	.0001
Sphincter of Oddi dysfunction	.00003
Staphylococcus aureus food poisoning	.0001

Stress gastritis	.001
Symptoms of chronic liver disease	.005
Systemic signs of pancreatitis	.004
Toxic megacolon	.00001
Tropical sprue	.000005
Ulcerative colitis	.0028
Upper GI bleeding	.001
Vipoma	.00001
Viral gastroenteritis	.005
Viral hepatitis syndrome	.002
Whipple's disease	.00001

GYNECOLOGICAL DISEASES

Abortion	.0012
Abortion; complete	.00024
Abortion; incomplete	.00065
Abortion; inevitable	.00012
Abortion; infected	.00001
Abortion; missed	.00001
Abortion; threatened	.0012
Anovulatory (dysfunctional uterine) bleeding	.01
At risk for ectopic pregnancy	.0001
At risk for pregnancy	.25
Atrophic vaginitis	.015
Breast abscess	.000003
Breast cancer	.00025
Cancer of the vulva	.00025
Cervical cancer	.0005
Cervical dysplasia	.01
Choriocarcinoma	.0000005
Dead fetus syndrome	.000064
Ectopic pregnancy	.0001
Endometrial cancer	.00002
Endometriosis	.0005
Fibrocystic breast disease	.08
Fibroid (uterine leiomyoma)	.05
First trimester pregnancy	.003
Gestational diabetes	.0009
HELLP (hemolysis, elevated liver enzymes, low platelets) pregnancy-induced HT syndrome	.000004
Hydatidiform mole	.000007
Iatrogenic postmenopausal bleeding	.0075
Leiomyosarcoma	.0005
Mastitis	.00006

Menopause	.35
Multiple gestation	.00009
Ovarian cancer	.0012
Pelvic findings of postmenopausal ovarian cancer	.0007
Pelvic findings of premenopausal ovarian cancer	.0002
Pelvic inflammatory disease	.001
Perimenopause	.09
Placenta abruptio	.00015
Placenta abruptio with fetal distress	.0004
Placenta previa	.004
Postpartum hemorrhage	.001
Preeclampsia	.0002
Pregnancy	.008
Pregnancy with Rh– mother and Rh+ father	.001
Premenstrual syndrome	.02
Vulvovaginitis	.003

HEMATOLOGICAL DISEASES

Acquired antithrombin III deficiency	.00001
Acquired platelet function defect	.005
Acquired risk of deep venous thrombosis	.05
Acute lymphocytic leukemia	.0001
Acute nonlymphocytic leukemia	.0003
Amyloidosis	.001
Anemia	.17
Anemia due to hemorrhage	.02
Anemia of B_{12} deficiency	.0003
Anemia of chronic disease	.02
Anemia of folate deficiency	.0003
Aplastic anemia	.000004
Cardiac amyloid	.0001
Chronic lymphocytic leukemia (CLL)	.00014
Chronic myelocytic leukemia (CML)	.00007
Clinical hemoglobin C	.0000002
Clinical thalassemia (major and minor)	.00011
CML in myeloblastic/lymphoblastic crisis	.000014
Cold hyperviscosity syndrome	.00005
Congenital antithrombin III deficiency	.0001
Congenital platelet function defect	.00001
Cyclic neutropenia	.0001
DIC (disseminated intravascular coagulation) (consumption coagulopathy)	.00003
Drug-induced immune thrombocytopenia	.0025
Drug-induced nonimmune thrombocytopenia	.0045

Enlarged spleen	.01
Evidence suggesting acute leukemia	.0004
Factor II (prothrombin) deficiency	.000002
Factor V deficiency	.000001
Factor VII deficiency	.000002
Factor X deficiency	.000002
Factor XI deficiency	.00001
Factor XII (Hageman factor) deficiency	.00001
Factor XIII deficiency	.000002
Gaucher's disease	.000002
GI manifestations of malabsorption	.001
Hairy cell leukemia	.0000032
Hemolytic anemia	.0019
Hemolytic anemia due to G6PD deficiency	.0011
Hemophilia	.00011
Hemophilia A (factor VIII deficiency)	.0001
Hemophilia B (factor IX deficiency)	.00001
Hereditary elliptocytosis	.0004
Hereditary ovalocytosis	.00004
Hereditary spherocytosis	.0008
Idiopathic aplastic anemia	.000002
Idiopathic thrombocytopenic purpura (ITP)	.001
Increased fibrinolytic activity	.0032
Infectious mononucleosis (CMV)	.000002
Infectious mononucleosis (EB)	.00017
Iron deficiency	.10
Iron deficiency anemi	.075
Isolated functional platelet defect	.001
Lupus anticoagulant	.0005
Macroglobulinemia of Waldenstrom	.00005
Methemoglobinemia due to cytochrome b5 deficiency	.000001
Methemoglobinemia due to hemoglobin M	.000001
Methemoglobinemia; acquired	.000008
Monoclonal gammopathy unknown significance	.035
Multiple myeloma	.0005
Myelodysplastic syndrome (refractory anemia)	.0001
Myelophthisic process	.0002
Myelophthisic process due to cancer	.00016
Myelophthisic process due to granuloma	.00002
Non-Hodgkin's lymphoma	.0007
Nonimmune hemolytic anemia caused by chemical or physical agents	.00078
Nonthermal hyperviscosity syndrome	.0002
Pancytopenia with hypocellular marrow	.000004
Paroxysmal nocturnal hemoglobinuria (PNH)	.00001

Pernicious anemia	.0004
Polycythemia	.02
Polycythemia due to high oxygen-affinity Hgb	.000001
Primary cryoglobulinemia	.000025
Primary fibrinolysis	.0002
Primary hyperviscosity syndrome	.00005
Primary myelofibrosis (agnogenic myeloid metaplasia)	.00002
Primary thrombocythemia	.00001
Relative ("spurious"; "Gaisbock's") polycythemia	.03
Risk factors for folate deficiency	.30
Secondary aplastic anemia	.000002
Secondary cryoglobulinemia	.000025
Secondary hyperviscosity syndrome	.00015
Secondary immune hemolytic anemia	.00065
Secondary systemic amyloid	.00002
Sensitized platelets	.002
Sickle cell anemia	.00004
Significant spherocytosis	.0004
Signs of abdominal lymphadenopathy	.01
Systemic amyloid	.00013
Thalassemia minor (alpha)	.0011
Thalassemia minor (beta)	.007
Von Willebrand's disease	.0002

INFECTIOUS DISEASES

Actinomycosis	.0000005
Acute HIV infection	.0001
AIDS	.001
AIDS-related Kaposi's sarcoma	.00003
Ascariasis	.00001
Aseptic meningitis	.00035
Asymptomatic HIV infection	.001
Atypical mycobacterial infection	.00003
Botulism	.000002
Brucellosis	.00001
Carbunculosis or furunculosis	.002
Cardiac manifestations of secondary Lyme disease	.05
Cellulitis	.004
Chancroid	.0001
Chlamydia; female	.0005
Chlamydial urethritis; male	.0005
Chronic symptomatic HIV infection (ARC)	.001
CMV (cytomegalovirus) in immunocompromised host	.0001
CMV pneumonia	.00012

CMV retinitis	.0003
Colorado tick fever	.00015
Constitutional manifestations of HIV infection	.001
Cryptosporidium enterocolitis	.0003
Culture-negative endocarditis	.0001
Cutaneous anthrax	.00001
Cutaneous leishmaniasis	.00001
Cysticercosis	.00001
Disseminated tuberculosis	.00005
Echinococcosis	.000001
Epiglottitis	.0001
Erysipelas	.0001
Erysipeloid	.000001
Esophagitis *Candida*	.001
Esophagitis CMV (cytomegalovirus)	.000045
Esophagitis herpes	.0001
Findings of bacterial infection	.05
Folliculitis	.005
Gas gangrene	.00001
Gonococcemia (disseminated)	.00005
Gonorrhea; female	.0005
Gonorrhea; male	.0005
Granuloma inguinale	.000001
Herpes genital (genital herpes simplex)	.005
Herpes simplex (herpes labialis)	.01
Herpes zoster	.005
Acute HIV infection	.0001
Hookworm infection	.00001
Impetigo	.003
Infective endocarditis	.0005
Inhalation anthrax	.000001
Legionella (Legionnaire's disease)	.00005
Lyme disease; primary	.0001
Lyme disease; secondary	.00006
Lyme disease; tertiary	.00003
Lymphogranuloma venereum	.000001
Malaria	.00006
Meningitis	.00001
Meningitis; cryptococcal	.00005
Meningitis; gram-negative (enteric/*Pseudomonas*)	.00002
Meningitis; *Haemophilus influenzae*	.0002
Meningitis; meningococcal	.00005
Meningitis; pneumococcal	.00015
Meningitis; staphylococcal	.00002
Meningitis; tuberculous	.00005

Mucocutaneous herpes simplex >5 weeks duration	.000036
Mucormycosis (zygomycosis)	.0001
Neurological manifestations of secondary Lyme disease	.10
Nocardia infection	.00002
Oral candidiasis (adult)	.001
Otitis externa; acute	.001
Otitis externa; chronic	.002
Otitis externa; malignant	.0005
Otitis media; acute	.01
Otitis media; chronic	.002
Peritoneal fluid findings of infection	.01
Peritonitis; dialysis-associated	.0002
Peritonitis; secondary	.0005
Peritonitis; spontaneous	.0002
Pharyngitis; gonococcal	.00003
Pharyngitis; streptococcal	.0033
Plague	.0000001
Pneumocystis carinii pneumonia	.00018
Primary lymphoma of the brain	.000003
Progressive multifocal leukoencephalopathy	.00001
Prostatitis; acute	.0002
Prostatitis; chronic	.005
Prostatitis; nonbacterial	.0005
Q fever (early)	.00003
Q fever (late)	.00001
Rickettsial encephalitis	.005
Rocky Mountain spotted fever	.000002
Sepsis	.001
Septic shock	.0025
Signs of acute HIV infection	.025
Sinusitis; acute	.005
Sinusitis; chronic	.01
Strongyloidosis; disseminated	.000001
Syphilis; primary	.00001
Syphilis; secondary	.0001
Syphilis; tertiary	.00005
Taenia saginata (beef tapeworm) infection	.00001
Taenia solium (pork tapeworm) infection	.00001
Tetanus	.0000001
Toxic shock syndrome	.00015
Toxocariasis	.00001
Toxoplasmosis in an immunocompromised host	.000024
Trichinosis	.00001
Tularemia	.00001

Viral URI (common cold)   .01
Visceral leishmaniasis   .00000001
Waterhouse–Friedrichson syndrome   .000001

NEUROLOGICAL DISEASES

Acute dystonic reaction   .00003
Acute subdural hematoma   .00025
Advanced sleep phase syndrome   .0001
Alcohol withdrawal state   .0005
Alcohol-dependent sleep disorder   .00025
Alcoholic polyneuropathy   .0005
Amyotrophic lateral sclerosis   .00001
Anterior inferior cerebellar artery syndrome   .00001
Arteriovenous malformation (cerebral)   .0003
Autonomic dysfunction of Guillain–Barre   .000005
Autonomic neuropathy   .0002
Becker's muscular dystrophy   .00003
Bell's palsy   .00023
Benign tremor   .02
Bilateral Bell's palsy   .000001
Blepharospasm   .00001
Brain tumor, supratentorial   .00046
Central pontine myelinolysis   .00025
Central sleep apnea   .0005
Cerebellopontine angle tumor (acoustic neuroma)   .00001
Cerebral abscess   .00001
Cerebral palsy   .0001
Cervical glioma   .00001
Cervical radiculopathy (C6/C7)   .005
Charcot–Marie–Tooth disease   .00004
Chronic inflammatory polyneuropathy   .0001
Chronic motor tic disorder   .01
Chronic subdural hematoma   .00006
Chronic time zone change syndrome   .01
Classical migraine headache   .01
Cluster headache   .0005
Common migraine headache   .05
Complicated alcohol abstinence (delirium tremens)   .0002
Concussion   .001
Cranial mononeuropathy VII   .0003
Creutzfeldt–Jakob disease   .000002
Delayed sleep phase syndrome   .005
Dementia due to metabolic causes   .0001

Diabetic neuropathy	.002
DOPA-responsive dystonia	.0000012
Drug-induced parkinsonism	.0002
Drug-induced tremor	.005
Duchenne's muscular dystrophy	.00015
Encephalitis (meningoencephalitis)	.00001
Epidural hematoma	.0001
Essential tremor	.03
Evidence of neurosyphilis	.00001
Evidence of syphilis infection	.0005
Facioscapulohumeral muscular dystrophy	.00005
Familial tremor	.01
Femoral nerve dysfunction	.00015
Frontal lobe hematoma	.002
General paresis	.000001
Generalized tonic–clonic seizure (grand mal)	.0002
Gilles de la Tourette syndrome	.002
Guillain–Barre syndrome	.00005
Hemorrhagic stroke	.0005
Hereditary spastic paraplegia	.00001
Huntington's disease	.00005
Hypertensive intracerebral hemorrhage	.001
Hypnotic-dependent sleep disorder	.0025
Idiopathic hypersomnia	.005
Idiopathic torsion dystonia	.000025
Increased intracranial pressure	.007
Intracerebral hemorrhage	.0005
Intraventricular hemorrhage (adult)	.000003
Irregular sleep-wake syndrome	.001
Isolated sleep paralysis	.00012
Lambert–Eaton syndrome	.00006
Left anterior cerebral artery syndrome	.00005
Left carotid artery syndrome	.00015
Left middle cerebral artery syndrome	.0005
Limb-girdle muscular dystrophy	.00001
Lower motor neuron syndrome	.001
Lumbar radiculopathy (S1)	.025
Manifestations of intracerebral bleeding	.002
Meniere's disease	.0001
Metastatic brain tumor	.0005
Metastatic extraparenchymal spinal cord tumor	.00001
Metastatic intraparenchymal spinal cord tumor	.00001
Migraine	.06
Motor dysfunctions associated with Guillain–Barre	.00001
Multi-infarct dementia	.001

Multiple sclerosis	.0005
Myasthenia gravis	.0001
Myelopathy (compressive); cervical	.0014
Myelopathy (compressive); thoracic	.0007
Myelopathy secondary to compression	.00001
Myotonic dystrophy	.0005
Natural short sleeper	.0001
Neurofibromatosis-1	.0003
Neurofibromatosis-2	.00003
Neurological signs of hepatic encephalopathy	.0004
Neurological findings of Sydenham's chorea	.000005
Neuropathy secondary to drugs	.00005
Neurosarcoidosis	.00003
Night terror	.003
Nocturnal paroxysmal dystonia	.00001
Non-24-hour sleep-wake disorder	.00001
Non-24-hour sleep-wake disorder	.00001
Normal pressure hydrocephalus (NPH)	.000012
Occupational (writer's) cramp	.00005
Olivopontocerebellar atrophy	.00001
Optic neuritis	.0003
Oromandibular dystonia	.000005
Parkinson's disease	.0025
Parkinsonism	.0026
Partial (focal) seizure	.01
Partial complex seizure	.005
Periodic limb movement disorder (PLMD)	.005
Petit mal seizure	.002
Pick's disease	.00001
Pituitary tumor	.002
Posterior cerebral artery syndrome	.0012
Primary brain tumor	.00005
Progressive supranuclear palsy	.000014
Pseudotumor cerebri	.00002
Psychophysiological (learned) insomnia	.005
REM-behavior disorder (rapid eye movement)	.0001
Repeated nightmares	.003
Respiratory muscle weakness-associated sleep disorder	.0005
Right anterior cerebral artery syndrome	.00005
Right carotid artery syndrome	.00015
Right middle cerebral artery syndrome	.0005
RLS (restless leg syndrome)	.005
Senile cerebral amyloid angiopathy	.00015
Senile dementia/Alzheimer's type	.0066
Sensory dysfunctions	.00002

Shift work sleep disorder	.02
Shy–Drager syndrome	.00005
Sleep eating disorder	.0001
Sleep state misperception	.00005
Sleep walking disorder (somnambulism)	.01
Spasmodic dysphonia	.00005
Spasmodic torticollis (cervical dystonia)	.00001
Stiff person syndrome	.00001
Stimulant-dependent sleep disorder	.0001
Striatonigral degeneration	.000025
Stroke	.005
Stroke secondary to atherosclerosis	.005
Stroke secondary to cardiogenic embolism	.003
Stroke secondary to carotid dissection	.0002
Stroke secondary to cocaine	.0001
Subacute combined degeneration	.00012
Subarachnoid hemorrhage (berry aneurysm)	.00011
Syphilitic aseptic meningitis	.000002
Syphilitic myelopathy	.000001
Tabes dorsalis	.000006
Tardive dyskinesia	.001
Tension headache	.01
Thalamic hemorrhage	.00025
Transient tic disorder	.015
Transverse myelitis	.00001
Trigeminal neuralgia	.0005
Vertebral/posterior inferior cerebellar artery syndrome	.0005
Wernicke–Korsakoff syndrome	.0005
Wilson's disease	.000001

PEDIATRIC DISEASES

Acute mastoiditis	.00001
Adducted great toe	.005
Alopecia trichotillomania	.0001
Bacterial tracheitis	.00001
Branchial cleft cyst	.00003
Breast milk jaundice	.0005
Breath-holding spell	.005
Bronchiolitis	.004
Cerumen obstruction/impaction	.003
Chicken pox	.002
Childhood volvulus (midgut volvulus)	.0001
Chronic dysfunctional stool retention in children	.003
Color blindness	.005

Congenital hip dysplasia	.0001
Congenital torticollis	.0001
Conjunctivitis; atopic	.001
Conjunctivitis; bacterial	.001
Conjunctivitis; viral	.001
Corneal abrasion	.0005
Croup (laryngotracheitis)	.006
Dacryostenosis (blocked tear duct)	.003
Diaper dermatitis; *Candida*-associated	.005
Diaper dermatitis; irritant-induced	.005
Discitis	.00005
Down syndrome	.0015
Encopresis related to stool retention	.00048
Enuresis	.001
Epstein's pearls	.005
Erythema infectiosum	.0005
Erythema toxicum	.005
Esotropia	.002
Exotropia	.001
Febrile seizure	.004
Foreign body in the ear	.0002
Fragile X syndrome	.0005
Gastrointestinal foreign body	.0002
Gastroschisis	.00017
Hand-foot-and-mouth disease	.0005
Head lice (*Pediculosis capitis*)	.001
Herpangina	.001
Herpes gingivostomatitis	.0001
Hirschsprung's disease (aganglionic megacolon)	.00003
Hypertrophic pyloric stenosis	.001
Infant colic	.0002
Inguinal hernia	.001
Inguinal hernia (infant)	.00012
Intussusception	.00017
Legg–Calve–Perthes disease	.00001
Measles (rubeola)	.0001
Medial femoral torsion	.0001
Medial tibial torsion	.001
Metatarsus adductus	.0007
Milia	.005
Miliaria crystallina	.0002
Miliaria rubra (prickly heat)	.0005
Mumps	.0005
Nasal foreign body	.0002
Neonatal clavicular fracture	.00005

Neonatal group B strep infection; early-onset	.00001
Neonatal respiratory distress syndrome (NRDS)	.00005
Nursemaid's elbow	.004
Omphalocele	.00008
Oral candidiasis (child)	.005
Orbital cellulitis	.00002
Pediatric asthma	.005
Pediatric dehydration	.001
Pediatric pneumonia	.005
Periorbital cellulitis	.0003
Peritonsillar abscess	.00001
Physiological jaundice of the newborn	.003
Pinworms	.001
Retropharyngeal abscess	.00001
Rhinitis; acute	.01
Roseola	.001
Rubella (German measles)	.00005
Scarlatina (scarlet fever)	.001
Sebaceous gland hyperplasia	.00125
Slipped capital femoral epiphysis	.00001
Spasmodic croup	.0006
Spinal muscular atrophy type I (Werdnig–Hoffman disease)	.000007
Spinal muscular atrophy juvenile type II (Kugelberg–Welander disease)	.000007
Stuttering	.01
Thyroglossal duct cyst	.0001
Toddler's diarrhea	.0015
Toxic synovitis	.00001
Tracheal or bronchial foreign body	.00003
Tracheoesophageal fistula	.00001
Traction alopecia	.03
Umbilical hernia	.018
Undescended testes	.0005

RESPIRATORY DISEASES

Acute bronchitis	.01
Acute mediastinitis	.00002
Acute mountain sickness	.0002
Acute pulmonary eosinophilia (Loeffler's syndrome)	.00005
Acute upper airway obstruction	.00001
Alpha-1-antitrypsin deficiency emphysema	.00011
Alveolar hypoventilation	.001

Asbestos-related pleural calcification	.00006
Asbestos-related pleural effusion	.00006
Asbestos-related pleural fibrosis	.00006
Asbestosis	.0004
Atypical pneumonia syndrome	.01
Berylliosis	.000001
Blastomycosis	.000001
Bronchial adenoma	.0002
Bronchial asthma	.05
Bronchiectasis	.0009
Bronchiolitis obliterans with organizing pneumonia (BOOP)	.00001
Bronchiolitis obliterans without organizing pneumonia	.00001
Caplan's syndrome (rheumatoid pneumoconiosis)	.00001
Chlamydial pneumonia (psittacosis)	.000001
Chronic bronchitis	.002
Chronic eosinophilic pneumonia	.00001
Chronic respiratory failure	.005
Chylothorax	.00001
Clinical manifestations of emphysema	.005
Coal workers' pneumoconiosis	.00001
Coccidiomycosis; acute (primary) pulmonary	.00001
Coccidiomycosis; chronic pulmonary	.00001
Coccidiomycosis; disseminated	.000001
Cor pulmonale	.001
CXR pattern consistent with primary lung cancer	.005
Cystic fibrosis	.0005
Diaphragm paralysis (bilateral)	.000001
Diaphragm paralysis (unilateral)	.00001
Diffuse interstitial pulmonary fibrosis	.001
Drug-induced pulmonary disease	.001
Emphysema	.0042
Empyema	.000033
Erythema nodosum	.00125
Evidence of mediastinal shift	.001
Fibrothorax	.00002
Flail chest	.00001
Goodpasture's syndrome	.00001
Hemothorax	.00015
Histoplasmosis; acute (primary) pulmonary	.000001
Histoplasmosis; chronic pulmonary	.000005
Histoplasmosis; disseminated (progressive)	.0000001
Hospital-acquired pneumonia	.01
Hypersensitivity pneumonitis (allergic alveolitis)	.0001

Idiopathic pulmonary hemosiderosis (adult)	.00001
Industrial bronchitis	.0014
Influenza	.002
Kyphoscoliosis lung disease	.00005
Lupus pneumonitis	.0001
Lymphomatoid granulomatosis	.000001
Mediastinal emphysema (pneumomediastinum)	.00004
Mediastinal fibrosis (granulomatous mediastinitis)	.000001
Mesothelioma (benign-fibrous)	.000005
Mesothelioma (malignant)	.00005
Metastatic cancer to the lung	.007
Metastatic pleural tumor	.001
Mycoplasma pneumonia	.0013
Necrotizing pneumonia (pneumonia with lung abscess)	.0005
Neurological manifestations of sarcoidosis	.00002
Noncardiogenic pulmonary edema	.001
Obesity hypoventilation syndrome (Pickwickian syndrome)	.00005
Obstructive sleep apnea	.005
Occupational asthma	.00015
Pleurisy (pleuritis)	.01
Pneumonia	.01
Pneumonia in immunocompromised host	.0025
Pneumothorax	.005
Primary lung cancer	.001
Primary pulmonary hypertension	.0001
Pulmonary actinomycosis	.0000005
Pulmonary alveolar proteinosis	.000005
Pulmonary aspergilloma (mycetoma)	.000001
Pulmonary aspergillosus; allergic bronchopulmonary type	.00008
Pulmonary aspergillosus; invasive type	.00005
Pulmonary AV fistula	.0000001
Pulmonary embolus	.001
Pulmonary function abnormalities of emphysema	.009
Pulmonary histiocytosis X (eosinophilic granuloma)	.0001
Pulmonary lymphangioleiomyomatosis	.00001
Pulmonary nocardiosis	.0001
Pulmonary systemic lupus erythematosus	.0005
Pulmonary tuberculosis (TB)	.00025
Pulmonary venoocclusive disease	.000001
Rheumatoid lung disease	.0001
Risk factors for TB	.35
Sarcoidosis	.0004
Signs and symptoms of pulmonary alveolar proteinosis	.001

Signs of increased ventilatory drive ("respiratory")   .0001
Silicosis (classical)   .0005
Silicosis; acute   .00001
Silo filler's disease   .00001
Solitary pulmonary nodule (benign)   .002
Solitary pulmonary nodule (malignant)   .0001
Spontaneous pneumothorax   .0025
Superior vena cava syndrome   .00001
Tension pneumothorax   .0001
Traumatic pneumothorax   .0025
Tuberculous pleural effusion   .00005
Viral pneumonia   .005
Wegener's granulomatosis   .00001

GENITOURINARY DISEASES

Acquired cystic disease   .00002
Acute bilateral obstructive uropathy   .0005
Acute interstitial nephritis caused by NSAIDs   .0001
Acute interstitial nephritis not NSAID-related   .0001
Acute nephritic syndrome   .0011
Acute renal failure   .0067
Acute tubular necrosis   .0002
Acute uncomplicated pyelonephritis   .0005
Acute unilateral obstructive uropathy   .001
Alport syndrome   .0002
Analgesic nephropathy   .0001
Anemia compatible with chronic renal failure   .05
Asymptomatic bacteriuria   .01
At risk for renal atheroemboli   .01
Atheroembolic renal disease   .0004
Bilateral hydronephrosis   .005
Carcinoma of the renal pelvis or ureter   .000075
Catheter-associated UTI   .0001
Chronic bilateral obstructive uropathy   .001
Chronic glomerulonephritis   .00093
Chronic renal failure   .0037
Chronic unilateral obstructive uropathy   .005
Complicated UTI ("chronic pyelonephritis")   .0005
Cystitis; interstitial (Hunner's ulcer)   .0001
Cystitis; recurrent   .01
Diabetes insipidus; central   .0001
Diabetes insipidus; nephrogenic   .00005
Diabetes insipidus; nephrogenic (acquired)   .00005
Diabetes insipidus; nephrogenic (congenital)   .00005

Diabetic nephropathy/sclerosis	.002
End-stage renal disease	.002
Evidence of membranoproliferative GN	.0003
Focal segmental glomerulosclerosis	.00013
Hemodynamically induced renal failure	.0005
Hemolytic uremic syndrome	.0001
Hepatorenal syndrome	.00035
Hydrocele	.005
Hyperkalemia	.001
Hypernatremia	.001
Hyperphosphatemia	.005
Hypocalcemia	.002
Hypokalemia	.005
Hyponatremia	.01
IgA nephropathy (Berger's disease)	.001
IgM mesangial proliferative glomerulonephritis	.00003
Imaging shows urinary calculus	.005
Interstitial nephritis	.0001
Lab evidence of UTI	.05
Lupus nephritis	.0005
Malignant hypertension (arteriolar nephrosclerosis)	.001
Medullary cystic disease	.000025
Membranoproliferative GN I	.00025
Membranoproliferative GN II	.00006
Membranous nephropathy	.00019
Mild azotemia	.05
Minimal change disease	.00019
Moderate azotemia	.01
Nephrolithiasis	.0024
Nephrotic syndrome	.00075
Nonspecific manifestations of renal failure	.01
Obstructive uropathy	.0075
Polycystic kidney disease	.001
Poststreptococcal GN	.00002
Prerenal azotemia	.004
Pyuria	.10
Rapidly progressive (crescentic) glomerulonephritis	.00006
Reflux nephropathy	.0004
Renal cell carcinoma (hypernephroma)	.00075
Renal failure	.01
Renal manifestations of sarcoidosis	.00002
Renal or ureteric colic	.004
Renal papillary necrosis	.0002
Renal tubular acidosis; distal	.0001
Renal tubular acidosis; proximal	.00002

Renal vein thrombosis   .00036
Renovascular hypertension (renal artery stenosis)   .001
Retroperitoneal fibrosis   .00005
Rhabdomyolysis   .0003
Severe azotemia   .005
Signs of inadequate peripheral circulation   .04
Testicular torsion   .0001
Transitional cell carcinoma of the bladder   .0015
Unilateral hydronephrosis   .01
Urinalysis evidence of glomerular disease   .003
Urinary culture positive for gram-negative rod   .30
Urinary culture positive for *Staphylococcus*   .10
Urinary tract clot   .001
Urinary tract infection (UTI)   .01
Urinary tract tumor   .002
Varicocele   .01
Vesicoureteric reflux   .001
Visible hematuria   .007

MUSCULOSKELETAL DISEASES

Achilles tendonitis   .004
ACL (anterior cruciate ligament) injury   .004
Acute gouty arthritis   .002
Adhesive capsulitis   .002
Adult Still's   .0001
Ankle sprain   .02
Ankylosing spondylitis   .005
Arthritis distribution consistent with tertiary Lyme
   disease   .05
Arthritis distribution in acute gouty arthritis   .001
Arthritis distribution of acute pseudogout   .003
Arthritis distribution of chronic gouty arthritis   .001
Arthritis distribution of RA (rheumatoid arthritis)   .01
Arthritis distribution of Reiter's   .001
Arthritis distribution of SLE (systemic lupus
   erythematosus)   .01
Avascular (aseptic) necrosis   .001
Behcet's syndrome   .00005
Bicipital tendinitis   .001
Bursitis   .01
Calcific tendonitis   .002
Carpal tunnel syndrome   .01
Chondromalacia patellae   .005
Chronic gouty arthritis   .001

Chronic pseudogout arthritis	.05
Compression fractures of the back	.005
CREST syndrome	.00005
Dermatomyositis	.0001
Ehlers–Danlos syndrome (type unspecified)	.00002
Enteropathic arthropathy	.0012
Eosinophilic fasciitis	.00005
Features of psoriatic arthritis mutilans	.0005
Features of psoriatic asymmetric oligoarthritis	.007
Features of psoriatic DIP (distal interphalangeal) arthritis	.01
Features of psoriatic spondyloarthritis	.002
Features of psoriatic symmetrical polyarthritis	.01
Felty's syndrome	.0001
Fibrositis (fibromyalgia)	.005
Fungal arthritis; blastomycotic	.000001
Fungal arthritis; *Candida*	.000005
Fungal arthritis; coccidiodal	.000001
Fungal arthritis; sporotrichosis	.000001
Giant cell (temporal; cranial) arteritis	.001
Gonococcal arthritis	.0005
Henoch–Schonlein purpura	.0001
Herniated nucleus pulposus	.005
Hypertrophic osteoarthropathy	.0001
Joint inflammation consistent with RA	.01
Joint pain consistent with monoarticular RA	.002
Joint pain consistent with polyarticular RA	.008
Juvenile RA; pauciarticular onset	.0003
Juvenile RA; polyarticular onset	.0005
Juvenile RA; systemic onset	.0002
Lateral epicondylitis/tennis elbow	.005
Lupus pericarditis	.003
Marfan's syndrome	.00004
Meniscus tears	.01
Necrotizing vasculitis	.0006
Neuropathic joint disease (Charcot joint)	.0001
Nongonococcal (septic) bacterial arthritis	.001
Osteoarthritis/DJD (degenerative joint disease)	.03
Osteogenesis imperfecta (type unspecified)	.00002
Osteomyelitis	.0005
Paget's disease	.001
PCL (posterior cruciate ligament) injury	.0004
Polymyalgia rheumatica	.002
Polymyositis (adult)	.0002
Pseudogout	.003

Psoriasis (plaque psoriasis)	.03
Raynaud's phenomenon	.002
Reflex sympathetic dystrophy	.001
Reiter's syndrome	.001
Relapsing polychondritis	.0001
Retrocalcaneal bursitis	.002
Rheumatic fever; adult	.0005
Rheumatic fever; child	.00001
Rheumatoid arthritis	.01
Rotator cuff tendinitis	.01
Scleroderma renal crisis	.000001
Sjogren syndrome	.001
Skin lesion of psoriasis	.02
Spinal stenosis	.001
Systemic lupus erythematosus (SLE)	.001
Systemic sclerosis (scleroderma)	.0001
Tuberculous arthritis	.0000025
Viral arthritis	.0001

Appendix 3
Using the Iliad KE Tool

In this chapter we will introduce a tool, called the **Iliad_KE_tool**, to help you construct an expert system.

1. Description of the KE Tools

The first step in knowledge engineering is the acquisition of knowledge from human experts, literature, and other references. The next step in the knowledge engineering process is using the KE tool to build the knowledge base. The "Iliad_KE_tool" is designed to meet this purpose. To construct the knowledge base, the "Iliad_KE_tool" facilitates the following steps:

1. Code the free-text terminology into the Knowledge Base Dictionary (Dictionary)
2. Create disease frames (Frame Author)
3. Build data relation files (Data Relations)
4. Build word relation files (Word Relations)
5. Provide precompilation checks (Utilities)
6. Compile disease frames (KB Compile) into the compiled object files (in the "Iliad Files" folder)

How to Begin

To run the "Iliad_KE_tool" and the "Iliad" program, you will probably want to create a new folder as a current folder (we use "KnowledgeEngineering" folder as an example in our book). Inside the current folder, you will need to put the "Iliad" program, the "Iliad_KE_tool" program, three dictionary files (DDcode, DDkey, DDtext), one or more subfolders containing frame author documents, two subfolders for relation files (DataRelations and

WordRelations), one subfolder for "Apriori Tables," one subfolder for "Picture Files," and one subfolder of "Iliad Files."

The "Iliad_KE_tool" will automatically create three DDfiles (DDcode, DDkey, and DDtext) at the first time when you open the program. If you run "Data Relation" and "Word Relation" functions, the "Iliad_KE_tool" will also create the "DataRelations" folder and the "WordRelations" folder for you. After you run the "KB Compile" function, the "Iliad_KE_tool" will create the "Iliad Files" folder. When you run the "Iliad" application, the program will create the "Apriori Tables" folder if you do not have one in your current folder.

2. Dictionary

To start the "Iliad_KE_tool" program, select (highlight) its icon on the desktop and either double click with the mouse or choose "Open" from the "File" menu.

New (Creating New Dictionary Files)

If you do not have the three dictionary files (DDcode, DDkey, and DDtext) in the current folder (such as the first time you begin to build your knowledge base), a window with the message "Can't open Dictionary Text file!?" may appear. Click on the "OK" button or hit the "Return" key. Then, you will see another window with the message "Do you want to create new dictionary files?" Click the "Yes" button or hit the "Return" key. The program creates new, empty "DDcode", "DDkey", "DDtext" files, and then automatically includes in these files several terms that are expected by Iliad to be in particular locations of any dictionary (i.e., age, sex, male, female).

If you want to create new dictionary files and you are already in the "Iliad_KE_tool" program, you first need to exit the "Iliad_KE_tool" program by pulling down the "File" menu and choose "Quit" or type "Command-Q". Remove the "DDcode", "DDkey", "DDtext" from the current folder. Then start the "Iliad_KE_tool" again.

List Dictionary Categories and All Items

The first time when you open the Iliad dictionary, you may want to look at what is already in the dictionary; or later, after you add some findings to the dictionary, you may want to look at all the dictionary items. To show all the first-level dictionary items (categories), pull down the "Dictionary" menu and choose "Root Levels" or type "Command-R" to list all the first-level findings [Iliad dictionary reserves the first level (L1) for general categories].

To display the children of a category, select (highlight) that category then double click it. Or, you can select (highlight) that category, pull down the "Dictionary" menu and choose "Show Children," or type "Command-Z." Either way will display all the immediate children of that category in "Dictionary Term" window.

Search Dictionary Items

Pull down the "Dictionary" menu and choose "Keyword/Code Search" or type "Command-K" to get the search definition window. Because each dictionary term is described with words (or keywords) as well as with 6-byte codes, there are two ways to search for finding(s): keyword search or code search.

To do the keyword(s) search, type in one or more keywords related to the concept word(s) and click in the "Search" button or hit the "Return" key. A "Dictionary Term" window will appear with the finding(s) corresponding to the keyword(s) you entered. Usually, a single keyword will retrieve a wider range of findings; multiple keywords will retrieve a narrower range of findings. It is not necessary to always use complete keywords for dictionary searching; you may only type in the beginning two (or more) characters of the keywords. Again, more characters will do a narrower searching and fewer characters will do wider searching.

If you know the code of the dictionary item, type in the code and click the "Search" button or hit the "Return" key. A "Dictionary Term" window will appear with the finding that matches the code you entered. If the search criterion is a code fragment, the "Iliad_KE_tool" program will assume the missing bytes are zeros. For example, a search for code fragment "1.1" is identical to searching for code "1.1.0.0.0.0" and both retrieve the term "General information." Separate your code numbers by either blank spaces or periods. If you search with a code fragment, you need to type in at least two characters (i.e., one number and one period or one number and one space) as the searching criteria.

All findings that match your keyword (or one finding that matches your code) are displayed on the screen in their hierarchical context (e.g., with parents). Each level of the hierarchy is indented to make the display easier to read. The "+" in front of a finding indicates that there is at least one finding further down this path in the tree.

Adding Dictionary Terms

There are three ways to add a new finding to the dictionary.

1. To add a new term at any desired place, pull down the "Dictionary" menu and choose "Add New Term."

2. To add a new term at the same level of an existed finding (level), select (highlight) that finding, pull down the "Dictionary" menu and choose "Add At Selected Level," or type "Command-A."

3. To add a new term below an existing finding, select (highlight) that finding, pull down the "Dictionary" menu and choose "Add Below Selected Level," or type "Command-B."

The "Editing" window will appear after you choose one of the three "Add" options. The "Editing" window for each of the "Add" menu options is the same except for the numbers in six boxes labeled L1 (level 1) through L6 (level 6) in the upper-left column. These boxes are for the six levels of the hierarchical code. "Add New Term" gives an "Editing" window with empty boxes. "Add At Selected Level" gives an "Editing" window with the code predefined as the next available code at the same level of your selected item. "Add Below Selected Level" gives an "Editing" window with the predefined code of the first available (unused) child of your selected item. However, you can always make changes to these predefined codes. The details of "Editing" window are described next.

Hierarchical Codes (L1, L2, L3, L4, L5, L6)

There are six boxes labeled L1 (level 1) through L6 (level 6) in the upper-left column of the "Editing" window. These are for the six levels of the hierarchical code. The code at each level is an integer greater than or equal to 1 and less than or equal to 255. In this hierarchical structure, you must add a parent level before you can add any children (e.g., add "Radiology" at level 1, then add "chest x-ray" at level 2 and "lung parenchymal abnormalities" at level 3).

In Iliad's hierarchical dictionary, the first level (L1) is reserved for general categories, indicating the source of information (e.g., Medical History, Physical Examination, Chemistry, Blood Bank, etc.). The second level (L2) is reserved for subcategories (e.g., type of examination performed, name of the test or procedure). For example, with Physical Exam data the level 2 terms include "vital signs," "abdominal palpation," etc. Iliad calculates the probability of a disease using the findings from levels 3 through 6 (L3, L4, L5, L6). Meaningful clinical terms are found at the third, fourth, fifth, and sixth levels.

Currently, L1 = 1 is reserved for Medical History, L1 = 1 and L2 = 1 is reserved for Demographic Information (or General Information such as age, sex, ancestry, etc.). L1 = 123 is reserved for decision frame titles.

The "Age", "Sex", "male", "female" are automatically included in the dictionary when you first create the new dictionary files. The code for "Age" is 1.1.2.0.0.0. The code for "Sex" is 1.1.8.0.0.0. The code for "male" is 1.1.8.1.0.0. The code for "female" is 1.1.8.2.0.0. Do not change these four codes; also, these four items need to be the first four findings in the Iliad dictionary. You can add any other findings anywhere after "Age" and "Sex: male, female."

As L1 = 1 and L2 = 1 (1.1.0.0.0.0) are reserved for Demographic Information (or general information), any finding under this subcategory could be treated as a risk finding (the disease will not be shown on a differential list if only these risk findings exist). Add the "real" findings (i.e., present illness of fever, physical exam shows heart murmur, or chest x-ray shows lung opacity) at the codes after L1 = 1 and L2 = 1 (i.e., L1 = 1 and L2 = 10).

Text

Each dictionary entry requires a text description. However, the actual text associated with a term is only a fragment of the full text that is displayed to the user in Iliad. Iliad requires only that each lower level in the hierarchy add a specific text modifier to the main concept. When the entry is displayed to the user, Iliad will concatenate all the text from this entry on up to the second level (L2) parent. For instance, the concatenated text "/Present history: /headache /pulsating /and unilateral/" is stored from L2 to L5. The text between "//" represents one level of hierarchical entry.

Type the text of your dictionary entry in the text box of the "Editing" window (i.e., cough). It is not necessary to end the text with a question mark because all items are presented to the user as questions. In the case of an item that requires a value answer, the text needs to contain three equal signs (===) as place holder for the result. Also, in the case of a value item it is necessary to indicate the normal values in parentheses at the end of the text [i.e., Serum potassium is === mEq/L (3.7–5.2)]. If you do not type in the normal value in parentheses, Iliad will assume the normal value is " =.0" (equals zero point zero) with one place of decimal point. When you answer a value question in Iliad, how many places of decimal point that Iliad could hold depends on the decimal point that you saved with normal value in the dictionary. For example, the normal range for blood pH is 7.35–7.45, so Iliad will hold two places of decimal point for it. The normal range for CSF red blood cell count is >5/μL, so Iliad only takes an integer for its value.

The item in square brackets [ ] will not be displayed in Iliad if the child of this item has been answered. For example, "/diarrhea /[quality] /[with mucus] /with blood-streaked mucus/" will be displayed as "diarrhea with blood-streaked mucus" in Iliad. But if "with blood-streaked mucus" has not been answered, Iliad will still display "diarrhea with mucus."

Keywords

The "Iliad_KE_tool" requires that each dictionary entry needs at least one keyword. Save keywords (for retrieving the term) by clicking the "Select Keyword" button in "Editing" window. All the meaningful words from the text will be inserted in the keywords box. Nondescript words such as "are", "as", "by", "of" etc. are discarded. You may type in additional keywords (such as synonyms or abbreviations) or delete any undesired keywords. Keywords can only be nine characters long, and the total number of keywords for each entry is limited to nine. If any keyword is longer than nine characters, the word is truncated (i.e., "examination" would be stored in the keyword file as "examinati").

Status

The status of a dictionary item refers to the type of answer or value that is associated with the item. Currently, the status is exhibited in two ways as "Yes/No" or "Value." For instance, the entry "fever" expects a "Yes/No" answer while the entry "Age" expects a "Value" for number of years. The default status assigned by the program is the "Yes/No" status.

Cost

Every item in the dictionary can have a cost value (but it is not required). The cost represents the dollar value of acquiring each piece of information. We suggest that you only give a cost to lab tests or procedures. The cost is an integer; no decimal point is allowed. The cost value is used by Iliad when ranking the cost-effectiveness of alternative diagnostic findings (e.g., choosing different lab tests or procedures for the same diagnosis).

The Flags

There are several flags in Iliad. The following flags need to be assigned in the "Editing" window.

The "**Chief Complaint Flag**" only applies to dictionary items that are current historical items the patient can provide, and Chief complaint is the problem(s) that brings the patient to hospital. This flag tells the Iliad simulator that the item can be selected as the presenting complaint of a simulated disease. The "Chief Complaint Flag" can be only used under code L1 = 1 (medical history). To assign a "Chief Complaint Flag," check the small box at left side of the words "Chief Complaint Flag."

The "**Not a Diagnosis**" (cluster) flag only applies to the frame titles (under L1 = 123). If a decision name is flagged as a cluster then Iliad will not include it as part of its main differential diagnosis list. This flag is used for intermediate decisions that are not top-level diagnoses. To assign a cluster flag to an intermediate decision, check the small box at the left side of the words "Not a Diagnosis."

The "**Non-Specific**" flag applies to an item that is not an answerable question. You do not want the user to answer the questions like "quality," "time pattern," "aggravated by," "relieved by" etc. Usually the not-answerable questions are at level 4 (L4) because the real findings start at level 3 and the level 4 is the group name for the modifiers. To sign the "Non-Specific" flag, check the small box at the left side of the words "Non-Specific."

The **Default 'No'** " flag applies to some parent items: if the user answers "yes" to one child, all the other children will be automatically inferred to "no" (e.g., if "Thyroid biopsy shows papillary carcinoma" is "yes" then "follicular cells" will be inferred to "no," "medullar carcinoma" will be inferred to "no," and "anaplastic carcinoma" will be inferred to "no," etc.), but you can always manually sign or change any inferred items to "yes."

Editing an Existing Item

To replace or change the text, code, keywords, or any item attributes (i.e., status, flags, frequency, etc.) in the dictionary, you need to search for that item first. Once you locate the item in the "Dictionary Terms" window, select (highlight) the item that you want to edit, pull down the "Dictionary" menu and choose "Edit Selected Term," or type "Command-E." The "Editing" window with all the information about the item will appear. Change any information you want to change, and then click the "Store" button or hit the "Return" key to save the changes. A window with the message "This will overwrite any existing record. Do you want to proceed?" will appear. Click the "OK" button to save the change; click the "Cancel" button or hit the "Return" key to go back to the "Editing" window.

Delete an Item

To delete a dictionary item, select (highlight) the item, pull down the "Dictionary" menu, and choose "Delete Selected Term" or type "Command-D." You can only delete the lowest level finding (the finding has no children under it). If the item you selected has a child, a window with the message "This term has children below. You can not delete it!" will appear. Click the "OK" button or hit the "Return" key. The item will not be deleted. Even if your selection has no children (the lowest level item in the hierarchical tree), the message, "Are you sure you want to delete this term?" will appear, and you will be asked to confirm your decision. Click the "Yes" button if you want to delete the item. Click "No" or hit the "Return" key if you do not want to delete the item.

Display

To display the children of a dictionary finding, you first select (highlight) the item with a "+" in front of it. Double click that item, or pull down the "Dictionary" menu and choose "Show Children," or type "Command-Z."

If the selected finding is collapsed, it will fully expand it (e.g., show all the children below). A subsequent double click (or pulling down the "Dictionary" menu and choosing "Hide Children" or typing "Command-Z) will collapse (hide) the lower nodes.

To see the numeric code of an item, you first select (highlight) the item. Pull down the "Dictionary" menu and choose "Hierarchical Code," or type "Command-H." A window will appear showing the 6-byte code of the item. Note: the offset value is for internal use; it indicates the location of the text in the DDtext file. The frequency is not used in the current version of Iliad.

In Iliad, the full text of a term is built by concatenating the text of each parent in the hierarchical tree. To show the complete text of a term, you can select (highlight) the term and choose "Concatenated Text" from the "Dictionary" menu or type "Command-T." A message window will display the concatenated text.

Statistics

If you want to know how many items are in the Iliad dictionary and how many items are in each categories, you can pull down the "Dictionary" menu and choose "Statistics." It only takes a few seconds to generate a report in a text file named "statistics.txt." The first column is the Iliad dictionary code from level 1 (i.e., "category 1" indicates L1 = 1; "category 2" indicates L1 = 2; etc.) and the second column is the number of the items in that category. The last line of the "statistics.txt" file is the summation of the items in the dictionary. The following is the example of the "statistics.txt" file:

category 1	2895
category 2	592
category 3	1149
category 4	225
total	4861

Export/Import Dictionary

You can create a text file version of the Iliad dictionary (including code, text, extra keywords, and other attributes). To do this, pull down the "Dictionary" menu and choose "Export Dictionary." Creating a dictionary text file may take a few minutes (depends on the size of the dictionary). A text file named "Dictionary.txt" will be created and saved in the same folder as the "Iliad_KE_tool" program. Exit the "Iliad_KE_tool" program. You can use any word processor program to open, format, and print the dictionary content. The following is the example of the dictionary text file:

1.0.0.0.0.0	History of present illness
1.40.0.0.0.0	Pulmonary symptoms:

1.40.2.0.0.0	wheezing ?c
1.40.2.20.0.0	[time pattern] ?s
1.40.2.20.2.0	nocturnal (worse at night) ?c
1.40.2.20.6.0	acute onset (5–10 minutes) ?c
1.40.2.20.8.0	onset at the age of ===
22.0.0.0.0.0	Hematological Lab Data IlaboratoryI blood testl
22.40.0.0.0.0	The bone marrow biopsy Ibxl {$150} ?n
22.40.2.0.0.0	shows normocellular
22.40.4.0.0.0	shows hypercellular Icellularityl
22.40.6.0.0.0	shows hypocellular
22.40.10.0.0.0	===% promyelocytes (1.0–8.0) Imyelocytel
22.40.16.0.0.0	===% lymphocytes (11.1–23.2)
22.40.20.0.0.0	=== % plasma cells (.0–2.0) Iplasmacytel
22.40.26.0.0.0	[shows blasts]
22.40.26.2.0.0	===% myeloblasts (.3–5.0)
22.40.26.4.0.0	===% lymphoblasts (≤.0) Ilymphocytel
22.40.26.6.0.0	===% monoblasts (.0–.8) Imonocytel
22.40.26.8.0.0	===% blasts (.0–6.0) Icelll
123.0.0.0.0.0	Diseases and intermediate decisions Iframe titles diagnosisl
123.142.0.0.0.0	Cardiovascular Ivascular cardiolog CVDI
123.142.3.0.0.0	Acute MI ICAD AMI myocardio infarctionl freq = .01
123.142.6.0.0.0	Pulse pressure ?d ?v
123.142.7.0.0.0	Signs of orthostatic hypotension Ibpl ?d

In this example, the very left column is the 6-byte code. The code numbers are separated by periods. The middle part is the dictionary text, additional keywords (which are not part of the main text), flags, and frequency. The text of the dictionary is indented by tab(s). First-level finding will have one tab between code and text. Second-level finding will have two tabs between code and text. . . . The main text, keyword, cost, and flags are separated by spaces. The frequency is the last part of a dictionary item, and is separated by a tab. The last line of the text is followed by a "Return" character. In the above example, there is a "Return" character after "Signs of orthostatic hypotension Ibpl ?d". The six byte codes and the dictionary text are the required two parts. All the attributes and additional keywords are optional. The following legend explains the symbols that have been used in the text version of the dictionary:

[ ]—This portion of the text is to be omitted by Frame Author and Iliad when a more specific node (a lower node) is displayed.

===—An item that accepts a value as opposed to a yes/no answer.

( )—For all value items, normal range are included in parentheses.

||—The words or characters between two vertical bars are extra keywords, which are not part of the text but is related to the main concept (i.e., synonyms or abbreviations).

{$}—Cost of each item

?c—A chief complaint flag (the problem that could bring patient to hospital).

?s—A nonspecific flag (for not a answerable question).

?n—A default "No" flag indicates that the parent item usually only has one child positive and all the others are negative by default.

?d—Not a Diagnosis flag. Decision is not a final diagnosis. This flag can only be used for frame titles (L1 = 123).

?v—A frame that returns a value. This flag can only be used for frame titles (L1 = 123) and a value frame is never been a final diagnosis frame (use "?d ?v" two flags together).

freq === frequency

You can also use the "Iliad_KE_tool" to convert a text version of dictionary to DDcode, DDkey, and DDtext format. To do this, follow the following steps:

1. Make sure the text file format is same as we have just described and the file type has been saved in "Text Only."
2. Check the desktop; the text file name must be "Newdictionary."
3. The "Newdictionary" file is in the same folder, at the same level of the "Iliad_KE_tool."
4. Open the "Iliad_KE_tool" program, pull down the "Dictionary" menu, and choose "Import Dictionary." A window with the message "Create dictionary files: NewDDtext, NewDDcode, NewDDkey from 'Newdictionary'" may appear. Click "OK" to continue.
5. You will see other three windows with the message "DDtext (or DDcode, DDkey) file already exists! Will create or overwrite NewDDtext." Click "OK" to each of these three windows. It takes a few minutes to create three DDfiles (depends on the size of the dictionary).
6. If there is a syntax error, a message window will appear to tell you what kind of error and where the error is located (line number or Iliad code).
7. Click "OK" and exit the "Iliad_KE_tool." Open the Newdictionary file and fix the error.
8. Do steps 4 and 5 again. If dictionary files have been successively created (no error message occurred), quit the program by pulling down the "File" menu and choosing "Quit."
9. Go to the desktop, remove the previous three DDfiles, and change the new DDfiles name from "newDDcode, newDDkey, newDDtext" to "DDcode, DDkey, DDtext."

The "Import/Export" functions are useful when the dictionary (three DDfiles) is damaged and you do not want to redo (reenter) the dictionary items again; you can use "Export" option to convert the three DDfiles to a text format, fix it, and then convert it back to DDfiles.

Print

Another advantage of exporting the dictionary to a text file is printing. You can print the complete dictionary (code, text, keyword, and other attributes) by using the "Export Dictionary" option (as we described in the previous section).

You can print only a section of the dictionary. To print only one branch of the hierarchy, first select (highlight) the item at the highest level of the branch you want to print. Pull down the "File" menu and choose "Print" or type "Command-P." A window with the message: "Print Keywords and Cost too?" will appear.

There are three choices: "Yes," "No," and "Cancel." If you only want to print the dictionary text with the corresponding code, click "No"; if you want to print the text, code, keywords, and cost, click "Yes" (this option takes longer); if you decide not to print, click "Cancel."

3. Frame Authoring

New Frame (Creating a New Frame)

To start authoring your frame, open the "Iliad_KE_tool" program (if it is not opened), pull down the "Frame Author" menu and choose "New Frame," or type "Command-N" to create a new empty frame. A list of all the disease categories that are in your Iliad dictionary will appear in a dialog window.

If no list appears then you need to "Cancel" the dialog, go back to the "Dictionary" menu, and add the category and frame title(s) in the dictionary (see Dictionary part, adding terms in the dictionary).

If there are more disease categories than will fit in the window, you can scroll the window up or down by clicking in the scroll bar at the right side of the window.

To select a category, move the cursor arrow over it and click. The category will be highlighted and the "Select" button at the bottom of the window will become active. Click the "Select" button or double click the category that you selected. A new dialog window containing all frame titles that have been entered in the dictionary for the selected category will appear.

If the title you are looking for does not appear then you need to "Cancel" the dialog, go back to "Dictionary" menu, and create your frame title.

Once again if all the disease names will not fit in the window, you can scroll through the list by clicking in the scroll bar at the right side of the window. Select the name of the frame you want to create by moving the cursor over it and clicking. The "Select" button will become active; click it or double click the frame title you selected.

Another dialog box will come up that requires you to choose the type of frame you will create: probabilistic, using Bayesian logic, or deterministic, using Boolean logic.

A Priori

If you choose probabilistic (by clicking the little button on the left side of the words "Probabilistic"), a box will appear asking for the "Apriori Value" of the frame. The "Apriori Value" must be a number between zero and one. For example, to create a new frame entitled "Acute_MI," choose the disease category "Cardiovascular." When the frame titles within cardiovascular appear, select "Acute_MI" as the frame you want to create. If it is a probabilistic (Bayesian) frame, click the "Probabilistic" button. Enter the "Apriori Value" into the box. In this example, it was entered with a value of 0.01. Click the "Done" button or hit the "Return" key; the "Apriori" value will then appear on the frame header window.

You can change the a priori value in a probabilistic frame anytime when the frame is open. To do this, select the frame header window (click anywhere inside of the frame header window), go to the "Frame Author" menu, and choose "Replace Apriori." A small "Apriori" window will appear, and the cursor will flash, waiting for you to enter a new value. After entering a new value, click the "Done" button. Your new value will be checked to make sure it is valid; then it will be placed in the frame header window. To cancel, clear the apriori box, and click the "Done" button; the original value will remain unchanged.

The Frame Header Information

The frame header information is now complete. The name on the top of the window is the frame name from the desktop. The first line of the header window tells you the category of the disease and the type of logic used by the frame (probabilistic or deterministic). The second line shows the frame title from the dictionary and whether the disease is a final diagnosis (Final Dx) or a intermediate decision (Intermediate Dx) that you defined in the dictionary. The third line shows the treatment threshold with a default value of 0.95 and the a priori probability. The last line contains the date and time of the last modification to the frame and the last date and time that the frame was compiled into the Iliad knowledge base. The modification date and time are updated whenever the frame is saved. The compile date and time are updated by the compiler when the frame is compiled. If the frame has not been saved, the modification date will be "New." If the frame has not been compiled, the compile date will be "Never."

Treatment Threshold

This number is only used if you plan to create simulations. The treatment threshold is a value set for each frame to signal the Iliad's simulator that a diagnosis has been reached. When the probability of a disease reaches its treatment threshold the diagnosis is considered to have been established with sufficient confidence to justify treatment. The Iliad simulator determines that you have solved the case when the data requested cause the probability of the correct diagnosis to exceed the preset treatment threshold.

When creating a new frame, the treatment threshold is automatically set to 0.95. You can change the treatment threshold any time the frame is open. To do that, select the frame header window (click anywhere inside of the frame header window), go to the "Frame Author" menu, and choose "Replace Treatment." A small "Treatment Threshold" window will appear with the current treatment threshold highlighted in the box. Type in your new treatment threshold, a number between zero and one, and click the "Done" button. The new value will replace the old in the frame header window. For most diseases, we use the default value (0.95) as the treatment threshold value.

Save Frame

You can save your frame any time when the frame is open. For saving a new frame, you need to make sure it will be saved in a subfolder that is at the same level of the "Iliad_KE_tool" program (inside the KnowledgeEngineering folder). To save a new frame into a subfolder, you need to pull down the "Frame Author" menu and choose "Save Frame As . . .". If the dialog window appears with a list of names in the "KnowledgeEngineering" folder, you need to either create a new folder or open an existing folder that is inside your current folder and save your new frame into the subfolder. To create a new folder, click the button with the word of "New." Another dialog box will appear.

Type the new folder name into the box below the words of "Name of new folder," click "Create" button or hit the "Return" key. Now, you are in the subfolder of the "KnowledgeEngineering" folder. Click the "Save" button or hit the "Return" key; your new frame will be saved in the new folder.

To save a new frame into an existing folder, pull down the "Frame Author" menu and choose "Save Frame As . . ." If the dialog window appears with a list of names in the "KnowledgeEngineering" folder, you need to select (highlight) the folder name which you want, double click it (or click the "Open" button) to open the subfolder, and then click the "Save" button. Your new frame will be saved in this existing folder.

To save a preexisting frame, pull down the "Frame Author" menu and choose "Save" or type "Command-S."

Open Frame (Opening an Existing Frame)

Pull down the "Frame Author" menu and choose "Open Frame" or type "Command-O" to open an existing frame. If the dialog window appears with a list of names in the "KnowledgeEngineering" folder (same level as the "Iliad_KE_tool" program), you need to select (highlight) the subfolder name that contains the frame which you want to open. If there are more names than will fit in the window, you can scroll the window up and down by clicking in the scroll bar at the right side of the dialog window. To select a folder, move the cursor arrow over it and click. The folder name will become highlighted. Click in the "Open" button or double click the mouse to open the selected folder. A list of all frame titles that are in the selected folder will appear in the dialog window. Once again, if there are more frame titles than will fit in the window, you can scroll the window up and down by clicking in the scroll bar at the right side of the frame names. Move the cursor arrow over the selected frame and click. The frame title will become highlighted. Click in the "Open" button or double click the mouse to open the selected frame.

You can also open a frame that is any place else on the disk. To do that, move the cursor arrow over the top center part of the window and press down the mouse. A list of parent folders all the way up the tree to the desktop will appear. As you hold the mouse down and move it up or down the different folders or desktop name will become highlighted. Letting go of the mouse will open whatever is highlighted. You can open any frame that appears in the window or continue searching the subfolders or parent folders as just described.

Frame Findings

To add, change, replace, or delete finding(s), you must first open the frame.

1. Add a finding

To add a finding to a frame, pull down the "Frame Author" menu and choose "Add Finding" or type "Command-F." The finding window will appear. This window is not the same for probabilistic and deterministic frames. For probabilistic frames you enter the keywords, the sensitivity, 1-specificity, and if your item requires, you can enter "If logic" or "Multiple bin" information. For deterministic frames you enter only keywords for the item. Entering keywords is the same for both probabilistic and deterministic frames. This section focuses on adding findings to probabilistic frames.

When the finding window first appears, the cursor will be blinking in the "Enter Finding" box. Enter any keywords for your finding that will later help you locate it in the dictionary. You are required to enter keywords (in the "Enter Finding" box), the sensitivity, and 1-specificity for each finding in probabilistic frames. To move the cursor between the boxes you can point and click with the mouse or use the "tab" key on the keyboard.

2. Sensitivity and 1-specificity

The sensitivity must be a number between zero and one. It represents the percentage of patients with the symptom in the disease population. The 1-specificity must also be a number between zero and one. It represents the percentage of patients with the symptom in the nondisease population. An item with sensitivity/1-specificity ratio >1 contributes positive information to the frame. An item with sensitivity/1-specificity ratio <1 contributes negative information to the frame.

3. If logic

Some findings, like many lab tests, need "if logic" to check for normal or abnormal values. To enter "if logic," click in the little box on the left side of the words "If Logic." A box will appear on the right, and the cursor will flash in the box, waiting for you to enter the logic.

When you click the "If Logic" check box, a "Help" button will also appear at the right side of the "If Logic" box. Clicking in the "Help" button brings up an explanation of "if logic."

4. Multiple bins

Some findings, like age, require multiple sensitivity and 1-specificity values that reflect the variance in likelihood ratio from an "age" range. To enter a finding with multiple bins, you need only enter the keywords and then click in the check box on the left side of the words "Multiple Bin." A new window will appear on top that allows for eight different results. The first column is labeled "Minimum." If the datum is greater than or equal to the minimum, value and less than the value of any next minimum, it falls into that bin and uses the corresponding "Sensitivity" and "1-Specificity" values. Use the tab key on the keyboard to move from box to box or point and click in the desired bin with the mouse. Enter the minimum value for each bin followed by the sensitivity and 1-specificity.

The following rules apply to the multiple bin:

1. The minimum can be any real number.
2. The sensitivity must be a number between zero and one.
3. The 1-specificity must be a number between zero and one.
4. The "Minimum" column must be in order lowest to highest.
5. If there is any input in a row, all three boxes in the row must be filled.
6. The "Clear" button at the bottom blanks out all the boxes in case you want to start over.
7. According to the information in the minimum column, we suggest that the number in the sensitivity column should add up to 1 and the number in the 1-specificity column should add up to 1.

After entering the multiple bin information, click "Done" or hit the return key to go back to the "Finding" window. The regular sensitivity and 1-specificity boxes will be invisible because you have entered them as multiple bins. The check box to the left of the words "Multiple Bin" will be checked to let you know that this is a multiple bin item. Clicking again on that check box will take you back to the "Multiple Bin" window when you want to change it. To delete a multiple bin, click on the check box and go back to the "Multiple Bin" window, click the "Clear" button, then click the "Done" button.

5. Risk factor

Some findings, e.g., "Hx of smoking," will increase the risk of a given disease but are not considered a manifestation of the disease. This is called a risk factor. Both probabilistic frames and deterministic frames can have findings with risk factor flags. To give a risk factor flag to a finding, click in the little button on the left side of the words "Risk Factor."

When all the information about the finding is entered, click the "Done" button in the Finding edit window or hit the "Return" key; this will take you back to the frame window. Every time the "Done" button is clicked. each field is checked for valid information. If something is invalid, the computer beeps and the bad item is highlighted while you are still in the finding edit window. Fix the invalid field, click the "Done" button again, and then go back to the frame window.

In the frame window, all the items in a frame are alphabetically labeled. Items that are preceded by an "*" are only keywords; they have not yet been mapped to the dictionary. An item associated with multiple bins or an item associated with "If logic" is a value finding. A finding with a "•" at the front is a cluster (frame). A finding with a "√" at the front is a risk factor finding. If there is "nor" or "xor" between two items, they represent an "or'd" group (the details are described in the following section).

6. "Or" groups

Often findings are related to one another in the context of a given disease profile (i.e., they are conditional dependent). Using more than one of these "conditional dependent" findings can cause Iliad to yield overconfident results in favor of a given disease. To deal with findings that are not independent of one another, we use one "or" the other (but not both) in Iliad's calculation of the posteriori probability. There are two kinds of "or's" in Iliad. One is "nor" (read as n or) the other is "xor" (read as x or). If all the findings are positive in the "or" group, the one that gets used is the one with the highest likelihood ratio (dividing the sensitivity value by the 1-specificity value). If some of the findings are positive and the others are negative within an "or" group, the "nor" and "xor" group will choose different finding for Iliad to use. The "nor" group always uses positive information (i.e., any positive overrides a negative). The "xor" group will choose the finding that contributes more information (i.e., stronger information overrides weaker information, either positive or negative).

To "or" two (or more) findings together, you need to select (highlight)
them. To do this, hold down the command key while clicking each finding.
When you have selected all the findings in the same group, then you go to
the "Frame Author" menu and choose "Assign NOR" (or type "Com-
mand-U") for "nor", or choose "Assign XOR" (or type "Command-V") for
"xor." The findings will be "or'd" and moved to the bottom of the frame.

You can "or" items either before mapping them to the dictionary or after
they have been mapped.

To remove the "nor" or "xor" from items in a frame, select (highlight)
any of the items in the "or'd" group and choose "Remove Or" from the
"Frame Author" menu or type "Command-M." The "nor" or "xor" from all
items in the group will be removed. If you want to change only part of the
"or'd" group, it is still necessary to remove the "or" and then assign them
again with your new group. To delete an item that is part of an "nor'd"
group or "xor'd" group, you must remove the "nor" or "xor" first. You will
then be allowed to delete the item. If you still want the rest of the items
from the group to be "nor'd" or "xor'd", it will be necessary to reassign the
"nor" or "xor."

7. Replace finding

To replace or change a finding in a frame, you must first select (highlight)
the finding. If a finding is too long to fit on one line, all lines will automatically highlight when you click on any one of them. Once the finding has
been highlighted, pull down the "Frame Author" menu and choose "Replace Finding" or type "Command-P." A "Finding" window will appear
with the current information displayed in each of the boxes. You can now
change or replace any of this finding's information the same as you would
when adding a new finding.

8. Delete finding

To delete a finding, you need to select (highlight) the finding, pull
down the "Frame Author" menu and choose "Delete Finding," or type
"Command-X."

Frame Logic

Deterministic (Boolean) frames require a logic statement in the "Logic"
window.

1. Add a logic statement

To add a logic statement to a deterministic frame, you need to select the
"Logic" window (to make it active) by moving the cursor arrow over the
"Logic" window and clicking it.

Then, pull down the "Frame Author" menu and choose "Edit Logic" or
type "Command-L." The "Enter Logic" window will appear.

There are two types of logic statements ("True If" and "Value If")
among the three kinds of deterministic frames. The three kinds of deterministic frames are described next.

The first kind is the most common one. The logic statement returns "true" or "false." When the "Enter Logic" window comes up, there is a default check (X) in the small box on the left side of the words "True if."

You are allowed to use only alphabetical labels of findings that have already been entered. For example, if you have two items, "A" and "B," you cannot say "A and B and C" because item "C" has not been defined. Click in the "Help" button for a description of valid "True if" statements. After entering the logic, click the "Done" button to return to the frame window.

During runtime, depending on the portion of the questions (findings) that have been answered, Iliad actually returns a percentage of closeness to true or closeness to false. Consider a frame with four findings, and the logic requires all of these four findings positive (A and B and C and D). If only two of the four findings are positive and we do not know, about the other two, Iliad then calculate the frame as being 50% true. This kind of logic allows Iliad to return **partial information**.

The second kind of deterministic frame returns a value; we call it "value frame." To change to the value deterministic frame, click in the little check box to the left of the words "Value if." You can tell which kind of deterministic frame you are in by which little check box has the "X." Type in the logic. This kind of value deterministic frame may do some arithmetic calculations and return the result (number). In the "Enter Logic" window, after you have checked the "Value if" box, you can click in the "Help" button for a description of valid "Value if" statements. After entering the logic, click the "Done" button to return to the frame window. If any parent frame use a value frame as a cluster, the higher level frame needs to contain a criteria in the "If logic."

The third kind of deterministic frame is also a value frame. You need to click on the little check box to the left of the words "Value if" to make it look like a value frame. However, it differs from the second kind of deterministic frame. This kind of frame can only return two values, 5 or 1. In this case, 5 represents "true" or "yes" and 1 represents "false" or "no." This kind of deterministic frame will **not** return partial information. In other word, it only returns 100% true or 100% false. The logic statement is just like a value frame, but the return value can only be 5 or 1. If any parent frame use this kind of deterministic frame as a cluster, the higher level frame needs to contain a criteria in the "If logic" (i.e., if item "A" is this kind of value frame, the "If logic" should be "A = 5" or "A = 1").

Your logic is checked each time the "Done" button is clicked to make sure it is valid. If something is invalid the computer will beep and the first unrecognizable character will be highlighted. If the logic is correct the frame window will appear on the top and the frame header will now say "Type: Deterministic (True)" for a "true/false" frame or "Type: Deterministic (Value)" for a value frame. The frame logic statements are only used with deterministic (Boolean) frames.

2. Replace or change a logic statement

To replace or change logic in a frame, you must first select (highlight) the logic. If the logic is too long to fit on one line, all lines will automatically highlight when you click on any one of them. Pull down the "Frame Author" menu and choose the "Edit Logic," or type "Command-L"; the "Enter Logic" window will appear with the current information displayed in the box. You can now change or replace any of the logic information the same as you would when adding new logic.

3. Delete a logic statement

To delete a logic statement, you must first select (highlight) the statement. If the statement is too long to fit on one line, all lines will automatically highlight when you click on any one of them. Pull down the "Frame Author" menu and choose the "Delete Logic."

Display Logic

The display logic is designed only for final diagnosis frame (both probabilistic and deterministic). Any top-level (final diagnosis) frame could have the display logic.

Usually Iliad will start to calculate the posteriori probability of a frame when it receives the first positive finding that is not a risk factor. However, if a frame has display logic, the Iliad program will first look at the display logic. If the display logic is not satisfied, Iliad will hold the posteriori probability in memory, but the frame will not be listed in differential window even if it is a top-level frame.

1. Add a display logic statement

To add display logic statement to a frame, you need to select the "Display Logic" window first (by moving the cursor arrow over the "Logic" window and clicking in it). Then you can pull down the "Frame Author" menu and choose "Edit Display Logic" or type "Command-G." The "Enter Logic" window will appear. Only use the default, "True if", for display logic; never use "Value if." Click the "Help" button for a description of valid "True if" statements. After entering the logic, click the "Done" button to return to the frame.

2. Replace or change a display logic statement

To replace or change a display logic statement, you must first select (highlight) the statement from the "Display Logic" window, then pull down the "Frame Author" menu and choose "Edit Display Logic" or type "Command-G". The "Enter Logic" window will appear with the current information displayed in the box. You can now change or replace any of the logic information the same as you would when adding new logic.

3. Delete a display logic statement

To delete a display logic statement, you must first select (highlight) the statement from the "Display Logic" window, then pull down the "Frame Author" menu and choose "Delete Display Logic."

Keyword to Dictionary Text

To link the keywords to Iliad's dictionary, you must first select (highlight) the finding, pull down the "Frame Author" menu and choose the "Keywords to Text," or double click on the finding with the mouse. The dictionary search window will appear with your keywords highlighted.

Click the "Search" button or hit "Return" to search the dictionary items that match your keywords. More keywords will give you a narrower search. Fewer keywords will give you a wider search.

The search can be limited by entering specific terms, but by using specific terms you risk the possibility that the finding in the dictionary was worded slightly different (e.g., pregnant and pregnancy). If that happens, type in more general keywords (or fewer characters) and search again. It is not necessary to type in completed keywords for dictionary searching. You may type in only the beginning two (or more) characters of the keywords. Again, more characters will provide narrower searching and fewer characters will do wider searching. You can also use the Iliad code to search if you know the code. To do that, highlight the keywords in the dictionary search window and hit the "Delete" key; then type your dictionary code in the search window. If you never find what you want, it will be necessary to go back the "Dictionary" menu and enter the finding in its proper hierarchical location in the dictionary and then map the frame item to it.

When you search the dictionary, all findings and their parents that match your keywords are displayed on the screen. Each level of the hierarchy is indented to help make it easier to follow. Findings with a "+" in front of them are parents. The "+" indicates that there is at least one finding further down the tree. You can expand and collapse findings with the "+" in front of them by pointing to the finding and double clicking with the mouse. When you locate the finding you are searching for, select (highlight) it and click the "Select" button. The keywords in the frame will be replaced by the text from the dictionary. The hierarchical code and attributes will be attached in the background to the item. The "*" in the frame for that item will disappear.

4. Relation Files

There are two kinds of relations in an Iliad knowledge base, "Word Relations" and "Data Relations." The first time you open the "Iliad_KE_tool," the program will create two subfolders, "WordRelations" and "DataRelations," in the current folder at the same level as the program.

Word Relation

Word relations help the user to do keywords search. For example: white blood cell, WBC, and leukocyte will be in one word relation group. When you search for white blood cell, you will get all the items with the keywords "white blood cell", "WBC," or "leukocyte." Word relations can be only one level or may span three levels of hierarchical context structure. For one-level-only word relation groups, you must have at least two keywords in the group (e.g., "biopsy" and "bx"). For two or three levels of hierarchical structure, you can have one or more keywords at each branch. For example, the first-level word relation has the keywords of "location, localized, area, where"; the second-level word relation has two branches, "distal" and "upper extremity"; "distal" is the only keyword in that branch. All keywords in one word relation group are displayed on the screen in their hierarchical context.

The following is an example:

Level	Text
	Level Text
0	location localized area where
1	distal
2	foot feet toe
2	hand finger
1	[upper extremity]
2	elbow
2	wrist

Here the number 0 indicates the first level, number 1 indicates the second level, and number 2 indicates the third level. The keywords in square brackets [] indicate that these two keywords always remain together like one word. When you do the search, you have to type "upper extremity" along with some other word in the relation group (do not need square brackets). Otherwise, you will get no response from this word relation. The reason for using the square brackets in this case is that we do not want to make "upper" and "extremity" as a same-level relation; in that case, when you searched for "extremity" you would get all findings that have "upper" in their keywords.

Add New Word Relation. Pull down the "Word Rel." menu and choose "New Relation." A window with the message "Please enter a title for this relation" will appear and the cursor will flash in the box (below the message) waiting for you to enter the title of this relation. Type in the title and click the "Done" button or hit the "Return" key.

You will see another window with the flashing cursor in the "Edit Text" box. Type in your first keyword (2 to 10 characters) and click in the "Add" button or hit the "Return" key. The keyword you just added will appear in the "Equivalent Terms" box (above the "Edit Text" box). The suffixes (such as -al, -er, -es, -ies, -d, -ed, -ion, -ation, -ing, etc.) will be truncated (e.g., extremity will be truncated to "extremit"). If you need to add more keywords at this level, type in the next keyword you want to add. To have a word relation group, you need at least two keywords in the same group.

Type two keywords together (e.g., upper extremity) in the "Edit Text" box, then click the "Add" button. These two keywords will be treated as one search term (they will appear in square brackets).

After you have added all the keywords at this level, click the "Done" button or hit the "Return" key. You will see the "Word Relation" window appear with the relation name on the top, three functional buttons (Change Relation Name, New Level Entry, Change Existing Entry), level indication at the left, and the keywords you just added.

You can add children to the parent level by selecting (highlighting) the parent-level keywords and clicking in the "New Level Entry" (check the level button at the left side of the window to make sure you choose the correct level); add new keywords in the "Edit Text" box (in the same way you would add the keywords to the first level). After you click the "Add" button, the "Word Relation" window will appear again. The level indication, at the left, tells you how many levels are in this word relation. The relation hierarchical context in the middle lists all the keywords that are indented by tabs. Each level of the hierarchy is indented to make the display easier to read.

When you finish adding a new word relation, pull down the "WordRelation" menu and choose "Close Relation." A window with the message "Do you want to save this file before closing" and three buttons will appear. Click "No" to exit the "Word Relation" without saving (you will lose your new word relation). Or, click "Yes" to save this new relation. Or, click "Cancel" to cancel the command (go back to the previous window).

Open Existing Word Relation. Pull down the "WordRelation" menu and choose "Open Relation." You will see the "Currently-saved Relations" window with all the word relation titles you have saved. Select (highlight) the relation title you want to view, and then click the "Select" button or double click the selected relation title. All keywords in that word relation group are displayed on the screen in their hierarchical context.

Change Existing Word Relation. You can change a relation title by first opening the relation and then clicking "Change Relation Name." You can change the existing keywords by selecting (highlighting) this keyword (all keywords will be selected at the same level) and clicking the "Change Existing Entry." All keywords you selected will be listed in the "Equivalent Terms" box. Move the cursor arrow over the keyword you want to change and click it only once (double clicking will delete this keyword). This keyword will be shown in the "Edit Text" box. Type the new keyword into the "Edit Text" box to replace the old keyword and click the "Change" button. Save the change by pulling down the "Word Relation" menu, choosing "Close Relation," and clicking the "Yes" button.

Delete Existing Word Relation. To delete an existing keyword, open that relation, click the "Change Existing Entry" button, then **double** click the keyword you want to delete (in the "Equivalent Terms" box). The keyword will disappear. Note: if you click the keyword (in the "Equivalent Terms" box) only once, this keyword will show up in the "Edit Text" box. But if you double click it, the keyword will be deleted. Save the changes as described previously.

Search with Word Relation. To search the word relation terms, you need to pull down the "Word Rel." menu and choose "Search Relations." A window will appear with the cursor blinking in the "Search Text" box. Type the keywords in the "Search Text" box and click the "Search" button or hit the "Return" key.

You can use word relations to help search Iliad dictionary items. To do that, pull down the "Dictionary" menu and choose "Keyword/Code Search" or type "Command-K"; to get the search definition window, check (X) in the little box on the left side of the words "Search w/Relation." Then type in your searching keywords in the search definition window.

The word relations will help you find findings when running the Iliad program. To run Iliad with the word relations, you need to have the "WordRelations" folder in your current folder ("KnowledgeEngineering" folder), at the same level as your Iliad program and the "Iliad files" folder. If the word relations folder is not in your current folder, each time when you open the Iliad program you will get a message, "Warning—The WordRelations are either incomplete or missing. Iliad can still run without them." The word relations will be used in Iliad "Keyword Entry" mode. You need to type in at least two keywords if you want to search with word relations.

Data Relation

Data Relations help Iliad to provide the "right questions" to the users. There are three types of Data relations: Not Applicable, Mutually Exclusive, and Same Value.

1. "Not Applicable" (N/A) relation lists all findings that should not apply to the category of that relation. For example, if the category is female, then the following findings are not applicable: (1) examination of male genitals; (2) history of prostatic disease; (3) prostatectomy; and (4) any other male problems. So, when you run Iliad, if the patient is a female, Iliad will not ask (omitted) these questions.

2. "Mutually Exclusive" (ME) relation groups several findings together. If one finding is "true" then all the other findings in the same group will be "false." In other words, if the user answered one question "yes," then all the other questions in the same "Mutually Exclusive" group will be inferred to

"No." For example, if the patient is a male then he cannot be a female. If blood group is A, then blood group is not B, AB, or O. If the patient has unintentional weight loss, then intentional weight loss and weight gain cannot be true at the same time.

3. "Same Value" (SV) relation gives an equivalent value to the other finding(s) in the same group. For example: "colonoscopy shows polyp" and "sigmoidoscopy shows polyp" need to be in one "Same Value" group; if one of these two findings is "true" then the other will be "true."

Create New Data Relation Files. If you do not have a "DataRelations" subfolder in your current folder or if you do not have an "notapp_file" inside the "DataRelations" folder (such as the first time you open the "Iliad_KE_tool"), you need to do the following:

Pull down the "Data Rel." menu and choose "Edit Data Rel."; the "Data Relation" window will appear. Select the type of the data relation from the three choices (Not Applicable, Mutually Exclusive, and Same Value) by clicking the small box to its left. After choosing the type of the data relation, all the buttons at the right side become active. Click the "New" button for adding a new group of data relation. If you do not have a subfolder named "DataRelations" at the same level as the "Iliad_KE_tool" program or if you do not have a file named "notapp_file" inside the "DataRelations" folder, a window will appear with the message: "DataRelations folder or notapp_file not found. Do you want to create them (one or both)?" Click the "Create" button to create the "DataRelations" folder and "notapp_file."

Add New Data Relation
1. To add a new "Not Applicable" relation, pull down the "Data Relation" menu and choose "Edit Data Rel." The "Data Relation" window will appear. Check (X) the small box at the left side of the words "Not Applicable" and click the "New" button; the "Search" window will appear and the cursor will flash, waiting for you to enter searching keywords. After entering the keyword(s), click the "Search" button or hit the "Return" key. A list of Iliad dictionary findings related to the keyword(s) you just entered will be displayed in the window below the search window.

Select (highlight) the item that you want; the "Select" button will become active. Click the "Select" button; a new, "N/A edit" window will appear. The first line of this window is the relation category that concatenates all the text from this item on up to the second-level (L2) parent. The findings listed below are the dictionary items that cannot apply to the category.

Clicking the "Add" button will bring up the "Search" window again. Type the keywords in the "Search" window and click the "Search" button or hit the "Return" key. A list of Iliad dictionary findings related to the keyword(s) you just entered will be displayed in the window below the search window. Select (highlight) the item you want and click the "Select" button. The selected dictionary item will be listed in the big box below the phrase "Not applicable To:" (that means this relation category is not applicable to the findings in the big box). You can add more items to this data relation group. When you finish with this group, click the "Save" button to save the relation that you just added and go back to the "Data Relations" window.

2. To add a new "Mutually Exclusive" relation, pull down the "Data Relation" menu and choose "Edit Data Rel." The "Data Relation" window will appear. Check (X) the small box at the left side of the words "Mutually Exclusive" and then click the "New" button. The "Mutually Exclusive edit" window will appear. Click the "Add" button; you will see the "Search" window. Type the keywords in the "Search" window and click the "Search" button or hit the "Return" key. A list of Iliad dictionary findings will be displayed in the window below the search window. Select (highlight) the item you want and click the "Select" button. The "Mutually Exclusive items" window will appear again with the finding that you just selected. You can click the "Add" button and add a new item to this relation repeatedly, or click the "Save" button to save the current relation and exit the "Mutually Exclusive items" window. You need at least two items in a "Mutually Exclusive" relation group.

3. To add a new "Same Value" relation, pull down the "Data Relation" menu and choose "Edit Data Rel." to open the "Data Relation" window. Check (X) the small box at the left side of the words "Same Value" and click the "New" button. The "Same Value items" window will appear. Use the same procedure as you would to add a new "Mutually Exclusive" relation and save it. Again, you need at least two items for each "Same Value" relation group.

Open Existing Data Relations. Pull down the "Data Relation" menu and choose "Edit Data Rel." to open the "Data Relation" window. Check (X) the small box at the left side to choose which type of relation you want to review. Click the "Open" button at the right side. A list of relation categories (for "Not Applicable") or a list of relation groups (for "Mutually Exclusive", or "Same Value") will appear in the next window. You can make changes (see following) to the opened relation. You can also review the hierarchy of the findings in any particular relation group. To do that, you need to select (highlight) the relation category (or group name) in the "List relation category" window (or "List relation group" window). Click the "Select" button; you will see the "Relation edit" window with the relation context of that relation group. Click in the "Expand" button; all findings will fully expand (e.g., show all the children below) and the "Expand" button will become the "Collapse" button. Clicking the "Collapse" button will collapse (hide) the lower nodes.

Change Existing Data Relations. To change, delete, or add more finding(s) to an existing relation, you need first to select the relation type and then open it. When the relation is opened, then do the following:

1. Not Applicable
   1. To review a relation, select (highlight) that relation category first. Click the "Select" button or hit the "Return" key; you will see a list of not applicable findings in the "N/A edit" window.
   2. To delete an N/A relation group, select (highlight) the relation category at the "List relation category" window, click the "Delete" button, and then click the "Done" button.
   3. To delete an item from its relation group, you need to get the "N/A edit" window, then select (highlight) the item that you want to delete, click the "Delete" button, and then save the change (by clicking the "Save" button").
   4. Adding a new item to an existing relation is the same as was described in the "Add New Relation" section.
2. Mutually Exclusive
Check (X) the "Mutually Exclusive" box and then click the "Open" button. A list of ME relation groups will appear.
   1. To review a relation group, select (highlight) a group name and click the "Select" button; you will see a list of findings that are mutually exclusive.
   2. To delete a ME relation group, select (highlight) the group name (e.g., "Group 1"), click the "Delete" button, and then click the "Done" button.
   3. To delete one item from a ME relation group, select (highlight) the item that you want to delete, click the "Delete" button, and then save the change (by clicking the "Save" button").
   4. To add a new item to the existing relation use the same procedure as was described in the "Add New Relation" section.
3. Same Value
Check (X) the "Same Value" box and then click the "Open" button. A list of SV relation group will appear.
   1. To review a SV relation group, select (highlight) a group name, click the "Select" button; you will see two or more findings that are equivalent or with same value.
   2. To delete a SV relation group, select (highlight) the group name (e.g., "Group 1"), click the "Delete" button, and then click the "Done" button.
   3. To delete one item from a SV relation group, select (highlight) the item that you want to delete, click the "Delete" button, and then save the change (by clicking the "Save" button).
   4. To add a new item to the existing relation, use the same procedure as was described in the "Add New Relation" section.

Search a Finding. To find out whether a finding is in a data relation and in what type of data relation, click the "Search" button. The "Search" window will appear. Type the keyword(s) in the "Search" box and click the "Search" button (or hit the "Return" key). The next window lists the finding that you selected. The left column with two characters indicates what type of data relation: "NA" means "Not Applicable"; "ME" means "Mutually Exclusive"; "SV" means "Same Value." You can review or change the relation from this window by selecting (highlight) the finding and clicking the "Select" button (or hit the "Return" key) to get the relation edit window.

Create Text Files. Click the "Create Text Files" button; the program will generate three text files for you to review. They are "NotApp.text" for "Not Applicable" relations, "MutualEx.text" for "Mutually Exclusive" relations, and "SameVal.text" for "Same Value" relations.

5. Knowledge Base Compile

The "KB Compile" option compiles the Iliad knowledge frames into binary object files that are used by the Iliad application program.

To run the "KB Compile" option, the three dictionary files (DDcode, DDkey, DDtext), Iliad knowledge frames folder(s), "DataRelations" folder (with the "notapp_file" inside), and the "Iliad_KE_tool" program must all be in the current folder. The frames in any subfolders of the current folder will be compiled.

There are three options in the "KB Compile" menu, "Compile All Frames," "Compile Subset Frames," and "Compile Relation." You will usually want to compile all frames, but for special purposes you can compile a subset of frames. To compile all frames, pull down the "KB Compile" menu and choose "Compile All Frames." It takes 1 minute to compile about 150 frames.

To compile a subset of frames, pull down the "KB Compile" menu and choose "Compile Subset Frames." A "Search" window will appear and the cursor will flash waiting for you to enter the searching keyword(s). Type the keyword(s) in the "Search" box and click the "Search" button or hit the "Return" key. A list of Iliad dictionary terms will appear in the big box below the "Search" box. You need to select a term (finding or frame title) from the dictionary and click the "Select" button. The "Search" window will appear again with the flash cursor in the "Search" box. If you want to compile more terms, type the next keywords in the "Search" box and click the "Search" button. After you select enough compiling items, click the "Cancel" button at the "Search" window. The program then compiles all frames that use the term(s) and any of its (their) child(ren) as well as all frames that are used as clusters inside any of those frames.

The "Compile Relation" option is used at the time when you change the "Data Relations" but have not changed Iliad dictionary and knowledge frames. To use the "Compile Relation" option, you must have the "Iliad Files" folder in your current folder.

If the "KB Compile" option encounters an error in any frame, that frame will be skipped. If more than 10 errors are found during a compile, the entire compile will stop and the errors will need to be corrected before you attempt to compile again. When errors are discovered, you will be told the nature of the error, which frame it appears in, and the number of the invalid item.

The "KB Compile" option builds 14 files and stores them in a subfolder called "Iliad Files" in the current folder.

6. Utilities

Pull down the "Utilities" menu and choose "Misc. Utilities." The "Iliad Utilities" window will appear. The options in "Iliad Utilities" are useful for checking Iliad source frames and the compiled Iliad knowledge base.

Select an option by clicking in the small circle to its left. Both the "Run" and "Explain" buttons will become active. Click the "Explain" button for a brief explanation of what the option does and what files are needed. Click the "Run" button to start running the selected option. Results are displayed on the screen. They can be printed and/or saved in a text file.

To run the "Utilities," the "Iliad_KE_tool" program and the three dictionary files (DDcode, DDkey, DDtext) must be in the same folder. Sometimes you will also need the subfolder(s) containing the source frames that you created with the "FrameAuthor" and/or the subfolder "Iliad Files" containing the compiled files created by the "KB Compile" during your last compile.

The source frames subfolder(s) are needed to run the following options: "Check Frames," "Find Finding," "Name and Title don't match," "Desktop to Dictionary Name," "Frames No Dictionary Title," "Multiple Frames Same Title," and "Change Frame Number (Title)." The "Iliad Files" subfolder should be in your current folder if you run the options of "Orphan Frames," "Missing Frames," "Top Level Frames," "Double Items," "Infinite Loop Check," "Compiled Frame List," "Levels of Nesting," or "Finding Occurrences."

Utility Options Available Before Compilation

Find Finding
This option asks you to select a finding from the dictionary, and then it searches for that finding in all the source frames. You can look for just that finding or that finding and all its children.

Check Frames

Before you compile your knowledge base, you need to run "Check Frames". Select the "Check Frames" option and click the "Run" button. It checks all your source frames (inside subfolder(s) of your current folder) for errors and omissions. It reports errors such as items not yet mapped to the dictionary, missing dictionary codes (codes of items that were mapped but the dictionary entry has since been deleted), findings expecting numerical answers but that have no threshold, logic statements that are invalid, etc.

Frames No Dictionary Title

This option lists all frames that have an undefined title. This can only happen if the title in the dictionary is deleted after the frame has been created.

Multiple Frames Same Title

This option checks all frames to make sure each frame title is unique. Multiple frames with the same code numbers will confuse Iliad. It is possible to have multiple frames on the desktop with different file names but with identical frame title codes. If multiple frames do exist that have the same frame title, they are displayed so you can get rid of the duplicates.

Name and Title Don't Match

This option compares each frame's desktop name to the internal (dictionary) frame title. If the two names are not the same, they are displayed.

Desktop to Dictionary Name

This option automatically changes all desktop frame names to match their internal (dictionary) name.

Change Frame Number (Title)

This option lets you choose any frame name from the desktop and then ask for the new title that you want from the Iliad dictionary. The code inside the frame is changed so that next time you read the frame it will have a new title. Also, the desktop name is changed to match the Iliad dictionary.

Utility Options Available After Compilation

Orphan Frames

Knowledge frames are either final diagnoses or intermediate decisions. Intermediate decision frames (clusters) are frames that are used by one or more final diagnosis frame. Because they do not stand alone, they must be called by another frame. This option checks for intermediate decision frames that are never called. They should be deleted from your knowledge base because they are only taking up space, or they should either be called by another frame or changed to become a final diagnosis.

Missing Frames

    Many times frames are used as clusters inside other frames. This option checks for frames that are called but do not exist. These missing frames must be found and compiled into the knowledge base or the reference to them by the calling frame must be deleted.

Top Level Frames

    This option creates a list of all final diagnosis frames.

Double Items

    This option displays dictionary findings that are used more than once in the same frame. Sometimes a frame will use the same finding more than once, but in such cases each occurrence of the finding will be looking for a numeric answer that falls in a different range. If a finding is used more than once in a frame and each occurrence is not checking for a value within different ranges, it is an error.

Appendix 4
Some Example "Domain-Specific" Symptom Lists

These lists can be used as picklists to facilitate quick data entry. No attempt was made to be complete in compiling the following lists. Only the major concept ("parent term") is included. Chest pain, for example, would also have numerous qualifiers for severity, time pattern, aggravating factors, relieving factors, etc. These "child terms" would be accessed on subsequent lists, dialog boxes, or forms. There are some symptoms that are suggestive of more than one specialty.

CARDIOLOGY

Hx of chest pain
Hx of chest tightness (dull pressure)
Hx of exercise intolerance
Hx of tachycardia (fast heart rate)
Hx of bradycardia (slow heart rate)
Hx of hypertension
Hx of palpitations (irregular or rapid heartbeat)
Hx of light-headedness
Hx of peripheral edema/swelling
Hx of shortness of breath
Hx of skipped heart beats
Hx of syncope

VASCULAR

Hx of a cystic mass
Hx of claudication (leg pain with exercise)
Hx of dependent redness of foot or extremity
Hx of aching in the calf
Hx of extremity pain

Hx of extremity swelling
Hx of mottling of the hand, foot, or extremity

DERMATOLOGY

Hx of a skin lesion
Hx of alopecia (hair loss)
Hx of bite (insect or animal)
Hx of dry skin
Hx of itching
Hx of nail abnormality
Hx of rash

ENDOCRINE/METABOLIC

Hx of amenorrhea
Hx of cold intolerance
Hx of defective sense of smell
Hx of dry hair
Hx of dry skin
Hx of episodes of lethargy
Hx of episodic sweating
Hx of fatigue
Hx of flushing
Hx of heat intolerance
Hx of impotence
Hx of increase in melanin pigmentation
Hx of increased appetite (polyphagia)
Hx of increased thirst (polydipsia)
Hx of increased urination (polyuria)
Hx of infertility
Hx of involuntary weight loss (>10% IBW)
Hx of irregular menses
Hx of lack of virilization at puberty
Hx of loss of libido
Hx of muscle stiffness (not rigidity)
Hx of muscle weakness
Hx of neonatal ambiguous genitalia
Hx of neonatal "salt losing"
Hx of obesity
Hx of pallor of rapid onset
Hx of palpitations of rapid onset
Hx of pelvic weakness (difficulty rising, climbing stairs, etc.)
Hx of secondary amenorrhea
Hx of short stature

Hx of sweating more than usual (diaphoresis)
Hx of tachycardia (heart rate >110)
Hx of tenderness or pain in front of neck
Hx of thyroid nodule
Hx of tremor
Hx of vitiligo (patchy skin depigmentation)
Hx of vomiting
Hx of weakness
Hx of weight gain >10 lb

GASTROENTEROLOGY

Hx of abdominal bloating
Hx of abdominal distension
Hx of abdominal pain
Hx of anal pain
Hx of anorexia
Hx of chest pain burning
Hx of constipation
Hx of diarrhea
Hx of dysphagia
Hx of early satiety
Hx of excessive flatus
Hx of excessive thirst
Hx of foreign body ingestion
Hx of generalized pruritis
Hx of hematochezia
Hx of hoarseness
Hx of jaundice
Hx of maroon stool
Hx of nausea
Hx of nausea and vomiting
Hx of odynophagia
Hx of pale stools
Hx of postprandial vomiting (several hours after meals)
Hx of regurgitation of food
Hx of scleral icterus
Hx of skin pigmentation increased
Hx of stool that is foul-smelling
Hx of stool with blood
Hx of stool with pale color
Hx of vomiting
Hx of weight loss (>10%)

GYNECOLOGY

Hx of being pregnant
Hx of breast tenderness

Hx of dyspareunia
Hx of edema
Hx of excessive menstrual vaginal bleeding
Hx of infertility
Hx of leukorrhea (vaginal discharge)
Hx of lump in breast
Hx of marked urgency incontinence
Hx of missed menstrual period
Hx of nausea/vomiting
Hx of nonmenstrual vaginal bleeding
Hx of painful breast
Hx of pelvic pain
Hx of pruritis of vulva
Hx of urinary burning
Hx of urinary frequency
Hx of vulvar irritation
hx of vaginal burning
hx of vaginal dryness
hx of vaginal itching

HEMATOLOGY

Hx of abnormal bleeding
Hx of bone pain
Hx of bone tenderness
Hx of easy bruising (ecchymosis)
Hx of fatigue
Hx of hematoma
Hx of involuntary weight loss
Hx of joint hemorrhage
Hx of pallor
Hx of petecchia and/or purpura
Hx of urticaria
Hx of WBC >15,000
Hx of weakness
Hx of weight loss >5%

INFECTIOUS DISEASE

Hx anorexia
Hx of a skin lesion
Hx of abdominal pain
Hx of back pain
Hx of chills
Hx of diarrhea
Hx of ear drainage

Hx of ear pain
Hx of facial pain over a sinus
Hx of fatigue
Hx of fever
Hx of headache
Hx of lymphadenopathy
Hx of muscle aches (myalgia)
Hx of nausea
Hx of painful skin lesion
Hx of passing worms in stool
Hx of sneezing
Hx of sore throat
Hx of stiff neck
Hx of vomiting

NEUROLOGY

Hx of abnormal involuntary movement
Hx of abnormal movements during sleep
Hx of sudden loss of visual acuity
Hx of anosmia
Hx of anxiety
Hx of arm weakness
Hx of bladder incontinence
Hx of blurred vision
Hx of bowel incontinence
Hx of burning pain
Hx of confusion
Hx of constipation
Hx of decreased ability to concentrate
Hx of decreased ability to maintain attention
Hx of decreased auditory acuity
Hx of decreased motivation
Hx of depression/dysphoria
Hx of deteriorating mood
Hx of difficulty ascending stairs
Hx of difficulty descending stairs
Hx of difficulty initiating sleep
Hx of difficulty maintaining sleep
Hx of difficulty running
Hx of difficulty swallowing
Hx of diminished alertness
Hx of disorientation
Hx of distal paresthesias
Hx of double vision

Hx of dry mouth
Hx of dysgeusia (impairment of taste)
Hx of dysphagia
Hx of episodes of paralysis occurring when awakening from sleep
Hx of excessive daytime sleepiness
Hx of face pain
Hx of facial drooping
Hx of fatigue, for weeks to months
Hx of seizure
Hx of footdrop
Hx of forearm numbness
Hx of gait ataxia (broad-based)
Hx of gait difficulty
Hx of having tics
Hx of headache
Hx of hearing loss
Hx of impotence
Hx of inability to lift arm above head
Hx of language disturbance
Hx of loss of abstraction
Hx of loss of consciousness
Hx of memory loss
Hx of muscle cramps
Hx of muscle spasms
Hx of muscle stiffness
Hx of numbness
Hx of paralysis
Hx of paraparesis
Hx of paresthesia
Hx of postural dizziness
Hx of seizure/spell
Hx of tinnitus
Hx of tremor
Hx of vertigo
Hx of visual disturbance
Hx of weakness
Hx of weak grip

OPHTHALMOLOGY

Hx of acute eye pain
Hx of acute eye redness
Hx of blurred vision of gradual onset
Hx of chemosis (conjunctival edema)
Hx of cloudy vision with halos, greatest in the evening

Hx of double vision
Hx of dry eyes (keratitis sicca)
Hx of excessive lacrimation (tearing)
Hx of excessive redness in the eye
Hx of eye burning
Hx of eye itching
Hx of eye redness
Hx of photophobia
Hx of red eye(s)

PULMONARY

Hx of cough
Hx of chest tightness
Hx of dysphagia
Hx of dysphonia
Hx of dyspnea
Hx of orthopnea
Hx of hemoptysis
Hx of chest pain
Hx of wheezing

GENITOURINARY

Hx of back pain
Hx of burning on urination
Hx of dark urine
Hx of flank pain
Hx of increased urinary frequency
Hx of nocturia
Hx of oliguria
Hx of polyuria
Hx of scrotal mass
Hx of suprapubic pain
Hx of urinary dribbling

MUSCULOSKELETAL

Hx of back pain
Hx of bone pain
Hx of extremity pain
Hx of joint pain
Hx of joint stiffness
Hx of joint swelling
Hx of knee catching
Hx of leg weakness
Hx of morning stiffness
Hx of pain in the extremities

Appendix 5
Example Data Relations

NOT APPLICABLE: In this list, within the same relation group, if the first finding is true then the following findings are not applicable (N/A).

Abdominal pain relieved by milk or antacids in a few minutes
  Abdominal pain aggravated by eating or drinking milk products
  Abdominal pain relieved by withdrawal of milk products

Current pregnancy
  Patient is null gravid
  Infertility
  Hysterectomy

Patient is null gravid
  Current pregnancy
  Pregnancy in the past
  Tubal pregnancy
  Termination of pregnancy
  Childbirth in the present or past
  Abnormal vaginal bleeding during pregnancy
  Abdominal ultrasound shows pregnancy
  Liver biopsy shows fatty liver of pregnancy (microvesicular fat)

Abdominal surgery: splenectomy
  Abdominal palpation: splenomegaly
  Chest x-ray (PA view) shows enlarged spleen
  Abdominal ultrasound shows enlarged spleen
  Isotope study shows spleen area increased
  Abdominal CT scan shows spleen abnormality
  MRI of abdomen shows spleen abnormality

Abdominal surgery: cholecystectomy
  Abdominal palpation: palpable gallbladder (Courvoisier sign)
  Abdominal film shows calcified stone in RUQ

Oral cholecystogram shows gallstones in the gallbladder
Abdominal CT scan shows thickened gallbladder wall
Abdominal CT scan shows cholecystitis
Abdominal ultrasound shows stones in gall bladder
Abdominal ultrasound shows thickening of the gallbladder wall
Abdominal ultrasound shows cholecystitis
ERCP shows gallstones
Radionuclide gallbladder scan

Female pelvic examination: undeveloped (prepubertal) genitalia
Female pelvic examination: cervix is moderately effaced
Female pelvic examination: cervix is dilated
Female pelvic examination: fetal membranes at cervical os
Abdominal ultrasound shows pregnancy
Female pelvic examination: retained placenta in uterus

Gender: male
Obstetric and gynecological history:
Headache aggravated by menstrual period
Abdominal pain during menstruation (dysmenorrhea)
Passing bloody or dark stool aggravated by menstruation
Pelvic pain began shortly after cessation of menses
Sexual dysfunction or hypoactive dyspareunia
Sexually active use of contraceptive vaginal diaphragm
Sexually active use of contraceptive oral contraceptive
Sexually active use of contraceptive spermicides
Sexually active use of contraceptive IUD (intrauterine device)
Sexually active use of contraceptive barrier contraception
Sexually active use of contraceptive Norplant
Past Hx of ob/gyn diseases
Examination of the breast: breast tenderness (mastalgia)
Female pelvic examination:
Ob/Gyn lab tests:
Serum testosterone === ng/dL for female (25–95)
Serum estradiol === pg/mL for female early follicular phase (30–100)
Serum estradiol === pg/mL for female late follicular phase (100–400)
Urine beta-HCG test (qualitative)
Qualitative serum beta-HCG
Quantitative serum beta-HCG
Serum FSH === IU/mL (1.3–6.3)
Hx of ob/gyn procedures:
Abdominal ultrasound shows pregnancy
Abdominal ultrasound shows abnormal adnexal
Abdominal ultrasound shows changes of uterus
Transvaginal ultrasound
Gynecological surgery

Exploratory laparotomy shows abnormality of the female reproductive
   system
Liver biopsy shows fatty liver of pregnancy (microvesicular fat)
Gram stain of vaginal discharge

Gender: female
Any male problems
Sexual dysfunction or hypoactive impotence
Itching on the inguinale
Injury or trauma to scrotum
Prostate abnormality
Serum testosterone === ng/dL for male (260–1100)
Serum estradiol === pg/mL for male (10–60)
Examination of male genitals:
Skin rash or lesion on penis
Skin rash or lesion on scrotum
Male genital procedures
Ultrasound of testis
Doppler of male genitourinary organs
Isotope study shows male genital abnormality
Transurethral prostatectomy
Prostatic cancer
Gynecomastia
Scrotal mass
Nonseminoma testicular tumor
Seminoma
Testicular dysfunction or failure
Epididymitis
Urology hydrocele
Testicular infection
Lesch–Nyhan syndrome

MUTUALLY EXCLUSIVE
Sex (male)
Sex (female)

Weight loss, unintentional
Weight loss, intentional
Weight gain, unintentional

Diabetes mellitus type 1
Diabetes mellitus type 2

Obesity
Emaciation or inanition or malnutrition

Joint pain acute onset
Joint pain insidious onset

Eye discharge
Dry eyes

Renal biopsy shows normal kidney by light microscopy
Renal biopsy shows renal cell carcinoma
Renal biopsy shows cystic disease
Renal biopsy shows glomerular disease
Renal biopsy shows interstitial disease
Renal biopsy shows vascular disease
Renal biopsy shows granulomas
Renal biopsy shows changes of multiple myeloma

Open lung biopsy shows bronchiolitis fibrosa obliterans without
   organizing pneumonia
Open lung biopsy shows bronchiolitis fibrosa obliterans with organizing
   pneumonia

Abdominal auscultation: hypoactive bowel sounds
Abdominal auscultation: borborygmus (hyperactive bowel sounds)
Abdominal auscultation: absent of bowel sounds
Abdominal auscultation: high-pitched rushing bowel sounds
Abdominal auscultation: absent of bowel sounds

Low-grade fever (101°F or 38°C or lower)
High-grade fever (102°F or 38.5°C or higher)

Skin rash or lesion unilateral
Skin rash or lesion bilateral

Skin rash or lesion began sudden or rapid onset
Skin rash or lesion began slowly or gradually

Blurred vision left eye only
Blurred vision right eye only
Blurred vision both eyes

Visual loss partially
Visual loss totally (blindness)

Cough with gross hemoptysis
Cough with blood-streaked sputum

Early childbearing (age <16)
Delayed child bearing (first child after age 30)

Delivery at full term
Premature birth (gestation <38 wks)

Abdominal surgery: partial gastrectomy
Abdominal surgery: total gastrectomy

Schizophrenia in one parent
Schizophrenia in both parents

Tall stature
Short stature

Examination of skin: single skin rash or lesion
Examination of skin: multiple skin rash or lesion

Ophthalmoscopy shows hard drusen
Ophthalmoscopy shows soft drusen

Ophthalmoscopy shows retinal hamartomas multiple
Ophthalmoscopy shows retinal hamartomas single

Otoscopy: normal auditory canal
Otoscopy: abnormal auditory canal

Examination of the nose: nasal septum is midline
Examination of the nose: nasal septum deviates

SAME VALUE

Chest pain aggravated by exercise
Chest pain relieved by rest

Foley catheterization gives relief of anuria
Retention of urine (not releasing urine from the bladder)

Abdominal distension
Distended abdomen
Excessive flatus
Distension with tympany

Echocardiography shows segmental left ventricular hypokinesis
Left ventricular angiography shows segmental hypokinesis
Echocardiography shows global left ventricular hypokinesis
Left ventricular angiography shows global hypokinesis

Colonoscopy shows polyp
Sigmoidoscopy shows polyp

Appendix 6
Example Word Relations

AAC
  antibiotic-associated colitis

AVM
  arteriovenous malformation

CNS
  central nervous system

GI
  gastrointestinal
  stomach
  duodenum
  bowel
  small bowel
  small intestine

HLA
  human leukocyte antigen

LMP
  last menstrual period

MAO
  monoamine oxidase

MCP
  metacarpal phalange
  metacarpal

MTP
  metatarsal phalange
  metatarsophalange
  metatarsal

PID
pelvic inflammatory disease

PIP
peripheral interphalangeal phalange
proximal interphalangeal joint
hand
finger

PVC
pulmonary venous congestion

STD
sexually transmitted disease
gonorrhea

AIDS
acquired immunodeficiency

SVCS
superior vena cava

TMJ
temporal mandibular joint

TURP
transurethral prostatectomy

ABDOMEN
abdomen
abdominal
belly
stomach

ABDOMINAL SERIES
KUB
flat plate
abdominal flat plate
abdominal series
kidney
ureter
bladder

ABDOMINAL SURGERY
bowel surgery
abdominal surgery

ABORTION
abort
miscarriage

ACHILLES REFLEX
ankle jerk

ACID FAST BACTERIA
  AFB
  acid-fast bacteria

ACID PHOSPHATASE LEUKOCYTE TARTRATE
  TRAP
  acid phosphatase
  leukocyte
  phosphatase leukocyte
  tartrate

ACIDOSIS
  pH
  acidemia

ACUTE LYMPHOCYTE LEUKEMIA
  ALL
  acute lymphocytic leukemia

AFFECT
  mood
  schizophrenia
  depression

AGGRAVATING
  aggravated
  exacerbated

AIDS
  HIV
  acquired immunodeficiency syndrome

AKINETIC
  adynamia
  hypokinetic

ALCOHOL
  ETOH
  ethanol
  alcoholic

ALKALOSIS
  alkalosis
  pH
  alkemia

ALPHA FETOPROTEIN
  AFP

AMEBIC
  amoeba

AMYOTROPHIC LATERAL SCLEROSIS
  ALS

ANERGY
  skin test

ANEURYSM
  aneurysm
  vascular ring

ANION
  anion
  Cl^-
  OH^-
  $HPO_3^=$
  $H_2PO_3^-$
  PO_4

ANOREXIA
  anorectic

ANTI-INFLAMMATORY
  NSAID
  nonsteroid antiinflammatory
  motrin
  ibuprofen
  naprosyn
  naproxyn
  indocin
  indomethacin
  felden
  piroxicam
  disalcid
  salsal

ANTIBODY HEPATITIS B SURFACE
  antiHBsAg
  HBsAg
  anti-hepatitis B
  hepatitis B surface antigen

ANTIGEN
  antigen
  Ag

ANTIMITOCHONDRIAL
  antimitochondrial antibody
  Ab
  antibody

ANTISMOOTH MUSCLE
  antismooth muscle antibody
  Ab
  antibody

ANTISTRIATED MUSCLE
  antistriated muscle antibody
  Ab
  antibody

ANTITHYROGLOBULIN
  antithyroid antibody
  thyroglobulin
  antithyroglobulin
  antibody
  Ab

ANXIETY
  anxious

AORTA
  aortic

AORTOGRAM
  aortograph

APPETITE
  hunger
  anorexia

APRESOLINE
  apresolin
  hydralazine

ARTERIAL CO$_2$
  pco$_2$
  pCO$_2$
  carbon dioxide

ASPIRATION
  needle aspirate

ASPIRATION PNEUMONIA
  necrotizing pneumonia
  lung abscess

ATAXIA
  ataxic

ATRIAL
  atrium

ATRIAL SEPTAL DEFECT
  ASD

ATRIOVENTRICULAR
  atrio-vent
  atrial ventricular

ATRIUM
  atrial

AUSCULTATE
  auscultation

AXILLA
  arm pit
  axillary

BACTERIA
  bacterium

BETA BLOCKER
  beta-blocker
  beta-adrenergic
  inderal
  propranol
  lopressor
  metoprolol
  tenormin
  atenolol

BILATERAL
  both sides
  symmetrical

BILIARY OBSTRUCTION
  bile duct
  chole

BIOPSY
  bx
  histology
  cytology

BLASTIC
  osteoblast
  normoblast
  monoblast
  lymphoblast

BLEEDING
  hematoma
  hemorrhagic diathesis
  blood disease
  coagulopathy

BLOOD
  blood
  serum
  plasma
  sera

BLOOD CELLS
  RBC
  WBC
  PLT
  red blood cell
  red cell
  erythrocyte
  white cell
  white blood cell
  leukocyte
  lymphocyte
  basophil
  eosinophil
  neutrophil
  poly
  monocyte
  PMN
  PML

BLOOD PRESSURE
  BP
  SBP
  DBP
  systolic
  diastolic

BLOOD UREA NITROGEN
  BUN
  serum urea nitrogen

BONE
  orth
  skeleton

BONE MARROW
  spinal cord

BOTULISM
  botulinum

BRAIN TUMOR
  glioblast
  astrocytoma
  oligodendrocytoma

    meningioma
    glioma
    medulloblastoma

BRONCHOGENIC CA
    bronchogenic carcinoma
    primary lung carcinoma
    primary lung cancer

BRONCHOSCOPIC BIOPSY
    bronchoscopy

BRUCELLA
    brucellosis

BULLOUS
    bullae

CALCIUM
    Ca^{++}
    Ca^{+2}

CALCULUS
    stone

CANCER
    mass
    neoplasm
    neoplastic
    tumor
    carcinoma
    sarcoma
    malignancy
    metastatic
    metastasis

CANDIDA
    candidiasis
    thrush

CARBON DIOXIDE
    CO_2
    carbon dioxide
    bicarbonate
    bicarb

CARDIOVASCULAR
    heart
    veins
    vessels
    vasculature
    cardio

CARPAL TUNNEL SYNDROME
  CTS

CEREBROSPINAL
  cerebrospinal fluid
  CSF
  spinal tap
  lumbar puncture
  LP

CHACHETIC
  cachexia
  emaciated

CHARACTER
  type
  attribute
  feature
  property
  quality
  description
  severe
  mild
  moderate
  sharp
  dull
  stabbing
  aching
  burn
  sting

CHEM 20
  chem-20
  smac20
  smac-20
  sma20
  sma-20

CHEM 7
  chem-7
  smac-7
  sma-7
  sma 7
  smac 7
  sma7
  smac7
  chem7

CHLORIDE
  Cl⁻
  hypochlorite

CHOLELITHIASIS
  gallstone

CHRONIC MYELOCYTIC LEUKEMIA
  CML

CHYLOUS
  milky

CLEOCIN
  clindamycin

CLONUS
  clonicity

COLOR
  black
  blue
  green
  cyano
  pink
  red
  white
  yellow

COPD
  chronic obstructive pulmonary disease
  chronic obstructive lung disease

COLD
  emphysema
  chronic bronchitis

CORNEA
  corneal

CORONARY ARTERY DISEASE
  CAD

CORONARY CATH
  heart cath
  coronary arteriography
  angiograph
  angiogram

COSTOVERTEBRAL ANGLE
  CVA

CREATININE
   creatine
   creatinin
   CK

CT SCAN
   comput tomography

CUBIC
   µl
   mm^3
   millimeter

CUSHINGS
   cushingoid

CYANOTIC
   cyanosis

CYSTIC FIBROSIS
   CF

DEEP VENOUS THROMB
   DVT

DELIRIUM
   delirious

DERMATOLOGY
   dermatitis
   skin
   cutaneous

DIABETES
   diabetic
   sugar
   diabetes mellitus
   glucose

DIABETIC KETOACIDIS
   DKA

DIALYSIS
   hemodialysis

DIGITAL PERIPHERAL
   DIP
   digital proximal
   digital phalange

DIGITALIS
   digoxin
   lanoxin
   digitoxin

DILANTIN
  phenytoin

DILITATION
  dilation
  ectasia

DIPSTICK
  dip stick
  multistick

DIRECT FLUORESCENT ANTIBODY
  DFA
  direct fluorescence antibody

DISEASES
  illness
  sick
  disorder

DISTENTION
  distended
  distension

DIVERTICULA
  diverticulosis

DROWSY
  hypersomnia
  somnolence
  sleepiness

DUODENAL
  duodenum

DURATION
  time
  length
  when
  onset
  begin
  began
  stop
  ceased
  lasting
  nocturnal
  sudden
  abrupt
  acute
  rapid
  slow

insidious
gradual
step wise
stepwise
chronic
prolong
morning
afternoon
evening
after
post
subsequent
before
previous
prior
past
during
last
lasting
post-prandial
postprandial
after food
after eating
after meal
preprandial
pre-prandial
intermittent
periodic
recurring
month
week
wks
year
day
min
sec
prodromal
sustain
prolonged
persistent
long
short
current
recent

exacerbate
paroxysmal

DYSPHAGIA
swallow

DYSPNEA, EXERTIONAL
DOE
shortness of breath
SOB

DYSPNEA, NOCTURNAL
PND

DYSTROPHY
dystrophic
dysplasia

EDEMA
swell
swollen

ELECTROCARDIOGRAM
ECG
EKG

ELECTROENCEPHALOGRAM
EEG

ELECTROLYTES
anion
cation
bicarbonate
HCO_3^-
calcium
Ca^{++}
chloride
Cl^-
magnesium
Mg^{++}
potassium
K^+
sodium
Na^+

ELECTROMYOGRAPHY
EMG

ELISA
enzyme-linked immunosorbent assay

EMBOLISM
  clot
  thrombos
  embolic

EMPLOYMENT
  worker
  employee
  occupation

END DIASTOLIC VOLUME
  EDV

ENDOSCOPY
  endoscopic
  scope
  fiberoptic
  colonoscopy
  EGD
  esophageal gastroduodenoscopy
  sigmoidoscopy
  anoscopy
  laparoscopy
  laryngoscopy

ENZYMES
  enz
  liver enz
  cardiac enz
  LFT
  pancreatic enz

EPISODES
  episodic
  attack
  exacerbation
  paroxysmal
  sudden onset

EPISTAXIS
  nose bleed

ESOPHAGEAL
  esophagus
  esophagoscopy

EXCISION
  resection
  removal

EXERCISE ECG
    stress test
    exercise test
    exercise ECG
    exercise EKG

EXPOSURE
    contact
    working
    occupation

EXTREMITIES
    distal
    peripheral
    upper
    lower
    extremity
    arm
    leg

EYELID
    eye lid

FAMILY
    brother
    children
    child
    cousin
    daughter
    family relation
    familial
    kinship
    father
    grandfather
    grandmother
    grandparent
    husband
    mother
    nephew
    niece
    parent
    sibling
    sister
    son
    spouse
    wife
    significant other

FARM
  farmer
  ranch
  agriculture

FARMER'S LUNG
  hypersensitivity pneumonitis

FATIGUE
  fatigueability
  tired
  prostrate
  lassitude
  malaise

FETUS
  fetal

FEVER
  febrile

FIBRIN SPLIT
  fibrin split product
  fibrinogen degradation product

FLUID LEVEL
  air fluid

FOOD
  eat
  meal
  diet
  milk
  dairy
  meat
  vegetable
  fruit

FOURTH
  4th

FRACTURE
  fx

FREQUENCY
  frequent
  interval
  rare
  recurrent
  repeat

FUNGAL
  fungus
  fungi

G6PD
  glucose-6-phosphate dehydrogenase

GALL BLADDER
  gallbladder
  bladder
  cholecyst
  gallstone
  gallbladder stone
  stone
  choledocho

GENITAL
  pubis
  testicle
  vulva
  vagina
  penis
  sex
  male
  female

GENTAMYCIN
  gentamicin
  aminoglycoside

GI HEMORRHAGE
  GI bleeding

GINGIVAL
  gum

GLAND
  thyroid
  adrenal
  parathyroid
  endo
  hormone
  pituitary

GLUCOSE
  sugar

GLUCOSE TOLERANCE TEST
  GTT

GONORRHEA
  STD
  gonococcal

GRANULOCYTOSIS
  granulocyte
  neutrophil
  WBC elevation

GROIN
  inguinal
  genital

GROSS
  massive

GUAIAC
  guiac

HEAD
  skull
  cranium

HEADACHE
  head ache

HEARING
  auditory
  aural
  deaf
  ear
  otic

HEART RATE
  bradycardia
  tachycardia

HEIGHT
  ht

HEMATACHEZIA
  feces
  gross blood
  stool

HEMATEMESIS
  vomit blood

HEMATOCRIT
  hematocrit
  VPRC

HEMOPHILUS INFLUENZA
  h-influenza
  h.influenza

   h-flu
   influenza
   hemophilus flu

HEPATITIS B SURFACE
   HBsAg

HEPATIC
   liver

HEPATOMEGALY
   enlarged liver

HISTORY
   hx

HORMONE
   ACTH
   ADH
   antidiuretic hormone
   AVP
   cortisol
   cortisone
   endocrine
   FSH
   gastrin
   GH
   GNRH
   gonadotropin
   growth hormone
   LH
   parathormone
   PLH
   prolactin
   thyrotropin releasing hormone
   thyroroid stimulating hormone
   TRH
   TSH
   vasopressin
   TSI
   renin
   angiotensin
   aldosterone
   estrogen
   estradiol
   progesterone
   testosterone
   HCG
   insulin

glucagon
erythropoietin

HYDROCHLOROTHIAZIDE
hctz
thiazide

HYDROXY
OH

HYPERCHROMIC
MCHC

HYPERGLYCEMIA
blood glucose

HYPERKINESIA
movement increased

HYPERLIPIDEMIA
triglycide
elevated lipid
cholesterol
LDL

HYPERMAGNESEMIA
magnesiume blood

HYPERNATREMIA
sodium blood

HYPERPHOSPHATEMIA
phosphate blood

HYPERREFLEXIA
reflex increase

HYPERTENSION
elevated blood pressure
high blood pressure

HYPERTROPHY
enlarged
increased size

HYPERURICEMIA
uric acid blood

HYPOALBUMINEMIA
decreased albumin

HYPOCHROMIC
MCHC

HYPOGLYCEMIA
blood glucose

HYPOKINESIA
  movement decreased

HYPOMAGNESEMIA
  magnesium blood

HYPONATREMIA
  sodium blood

HYPONEPHROMA
  renal cell carcinoma

HYPOPHOSPHATEMIA
  phosphate blood

HYPOREFLEXIA
  reflex decreased

HYPOURICEMIA
  uric acid blood

HYPOXEMIA
  oxygen tension blood
  oxygen saturation
  cyanosis

IMMOBILIZED
  immobilization
  immobile
  bed rest
  bedrest
  inactivity
  inactive

IMPULSE APICAL
  PMI

INFANT
  neonate
  neonatal
  newborn

INSOMNIA
  sleep difficulty

INTERSPACE BORDER
  sternal border
  ILSB
  fourth interspace border

INTRAUTERINE DEVICE
  IUD

INTRAVENOUS PYELOGRAM
  IVP

IODINE
   radioiodine
   contrast
   radiocontrast
   iodide

IPSILATERAL
   same side

IRON BINDING CAPACITY
   TIBC
   iron binding capacity
   total iron binding

ISONIAZID
   INH
   isoniazid

ITCH
   pruritis
   itchy

JAUNDICE
   icterus
   yellow skin

JOINT, ARTHRITIS
   arthralgia
   arthritis
   joint pain
   joint swelling
   joint stiffness

JOINT
   shoulder
   elbow
   wrist
   mcp
   hip
   knee patella
   ankle
   toe
   mtp
   dip
   pip

KETONE
   acetone
   ketonuria
   ketonemia

KYPOKALEMIA
  potassium blood
LACTATE DEHYDROGENASE
  LDH
LEFT
  unilateral
LEFT AXIS
  LAD
LEFT BUNDLE
  LBBB
LEFT HYPERTROPHIC
  LVH
LEGIONELLA
  legionaire
  legionnaire
  atypical pneumonia
LIBIDO
  sexual drive
  sex drive
  sexual desire
LICE
  louse
LINCOCIN
  lincomycin
LIPID
  fat
  lipo
LOCATION
  site
  local
  where
  localized
  diffuse
  area
  anterior
  posterior
  distal
  proximal
  upper
  lower
  right side
  left side

symmetrical
inferior
superior

LOWER ABDOMEN
suprapubic

LEUTINIZING HORMONE
LH

LYMPHOMA
mass
tumor
cancer
neoplasm

LYTIC
osteolytic

MACROCYTIC
MCV

MADE BETTER
improve
decrease
recover
relief
alleviate
assuage
diminish
mitigate

MADE WORSE
increase
amplify
exacerbate
intensify
augment
aggravate
magnify

MAGNESIUM
Mg^{++}
Mg^{+2}

MANOMETRY
manometric

MANY
multiple
a lot

MAXIMUM
  maximal
  maxim

MCG
  microgram
  μg

MEDICATION
  medicine
  drug
  pill

MENSTRUATION
  mense
  menstrual
  menarch
  menopause

MICROCYTIC
  MCV

MOTION
  movement

MOUTH
  oral
  buccal
  pharyngeal

MULTIPLE ENDOCRINE NEOPLASM
  MEN

MULTIPLE JOINTS
  polyarthritis

MYCETOMA
  fungal ball
  fungus ball

NECROTIC
  necrosis

NEUROFIBROMATOSIS
  NF

NEUTROPENIA
  neutrophil absent
  neutrophil decreased

NITROGLYCERIN
  NTG

NOCTURIA
  night urination

NODULES
  node
  nodular
  lymph node
  adenopathy
  lymphadeny
  lymph node enlargement
  cervical node
  axillary node
  inguinal node

OPHTHALMIC
  eye
  ocular
  optic

ORAL CHOLECYSTOGRAM
  OCG

OROMANDIBULAR
  oro mandibular

OSMOLARITY
  osmolar
  tonicity
  osmolality
  hyposmolar
  hyperosmolar
  normosmolar
  osmotic pressure

OTITIS MEDIA
  ear pain
  earache

OVERDOSE
  drug abuse

OXYGEN TENSION BLOOD
  pO_2
  blood tension

PAINFUL
  ache
  aching
  sore
  dolor
  hurt
  tender

PALLOR
  pale
PALPATION
  palpable
PANCREATIC
  pancreas
PARALYSIS
  palsy
  pares
  paralytic
  hemipares
  paraplegia
  quadraplegia
  flaccid
  weakness
  strength
PARENTERAL
  IV drug use
  drug administration
PARESTHESIA
  numbness
PARTIAL THROMBOPLASTIN TIME
  PTT
PATELLAR REFLEX
  knee jerk
PATENT DUCTUS ARTERIOSUS
  PDA
PHALLIC
  phallus
  penile
  penis
PHARYNGITIS
  sore throat
PHYSICAL EXAM
  PE
  sign
PODAGRE
  toe
POSTURE
  position
  lying

lie
sitting
sit
stand
supine
prone

POTASSIUM
K+

PREGNANCY
gravid
pregnant

PROTHESIS
prosthetic
artificial

PROTHROMBIN TIME
PT

PSYCHOSOCIAL
job loss
mental stress
financial difficulty
death of loved one

RADIATES
refer to

RADIOIOSOTOPE
thalium
scan
nucleid
hida
thyroid scan

REGION
area

RENAL
kidney
nephro

RESIDENCE
travel

RESPIRATION
breath
ventilation

RHEUMATOID ARTHRITIS
joint disease

RIGHT
  unilateral
  sidedness

RIGHT AXIS
  RAD

RIGHT BUNDLE
  RBBB

RUB
  friction rub
  crepitus

SCLERA
  scleral

SEASONAL
  season
  spring
  summer
  autumn
  fall
  winter

SECOND
  2nd

SEDIMENTATION RATE
  ESR
  sed rate
  sed-rate

SEIZURE
  fit
  seizing
  convulse
  convulsion
  seize

SEROLOGY
  seropositive
  precipitin
  PPT
  precipitation
  complement fixation
  immunoelectrophoresis
  immunofixation

SHORTNESS OF BREATH
  SOB
  dyspnea

breathless

SIZE
measure
dimension
length
width
small
big
large
medium
height
weight

SKIN
cutaneous
derm

SMEAR
stain

SODIUM
salt
Na^+

SPLENOMEGALY
enlarged spleen

SPURS
osteophyte

SPUTUM
productive cough

STAPHYLOCOCCUS
staphyloccal

STEROID
glucocorticoid
mineralocorticoid
aldosterone
corticosteroid
prednisone
solumedrol
cortisone
hydrocortisone
dexamethasone

STOOL
feces
fecal

STRABISMUS
  wander eye
  strabism
  extraocular muscle weakness
  muscle eye weakness

STREPTOCOCCUS
  streptoccal

STREPTOLYSIN O
  ASO

SURGERY
  surgical
  post op
  pre op
  pre-op
  post-op

SYNCOPE
  faint
  black out
  blackout
  dizzy
  stoke

SYNDROME INAPPROPRIATE ANTIDIURETIC HORMONE
  SIADH

SYNOVIUM
  synovial

SYSTEMIC LUPUS ERYTHEMATOSUS
  SLE

SYSTOLIC EJECT MURMUR
  SEM

SYSTOLIC
  holosystolic
  presystolic
  midsystolic

TACHYCARDIA
  heart rate increase

TACHYPNEA
  respiratory rate increase

TARSAL
  instep

TEARS
  lacrimal

TESTES
  testicle
  testicular

TESTOSTERONE
  androgen

THIRD
  3rd

THORACENTESIS
  pleural fluid

THROMBOCYTOSIS
  platelet increase

THYROID TESTS
  TFT
  T4
  T3U
  resin uptake
  T3
  FTI
  TSH
  thyroxin

THYROID, ENLARGED
  goiter
  thyroid enlargement

TINEA
  ringworm

TITERS
  titre

TOBRAMYCIN
  tobramicin
  aminoglycoside

TOMOGRAPHY
  CT

TOTAL LUNG CAPACITY
  TLC

TOUCH
  tactile

TUBERCULOSIS
  TB
  mycobacterium
  acid fast stain

TULAREMIA
  tularensis
TYLENOL
  acetaminophen
ULTRASOUND
  ultrasonography
UNILATERAL
  one side
  one-side
UPPER GI
  UGI
  barium
UPPER RESPIRATORY INFECTION
  URI
UREMIA
  azotemia
  urea
  blood nitrogen
URINARY TRACT INFECTION
  UTI
URINE
  urinary
  urination
  micturition
  void
  urinate
URINE OUTPUT
  oliguria
  polyuria
  anuria
VALSALVA
  squat
VALVE
  mitral
  tricuspid
VARICES
  varix
VENOGRAM
  venograph
VENTRICULAR PREMATURE CONTRACTIONS
  PVC
  VPC

VENTRICULAR SEPTAL DEFECT
  VSD
VENTRICULAR
  ventricle
VENTRICULAR FIBRILLATION
  vfib
  v fib
VESICULAR
  vesicle
VESSEL
  vascular
VIRUS
  viral
  EB
  CMV
  HBV
  HCV
  HAV
  HIV
VISION
  visual
  cataract
WHEEZE
  wheezing
XRAY
  x-ray
  x ray
  radiogram
  radiograph
  radiology
  film
  cxr
  chest xray
YEAR
  yrs
  year
  yr

Index